SLIM
FOR
LIFE

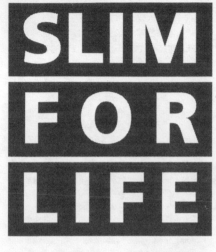

Judith Wills

ARROW

To Chris and William

First published in 1994

1 3 5 7 9 10 8 6 4 2

Copyright © Judith Wills 1994

First published in the United Kingdom in 1994
by Vermilion Arrow
an imprint of Ebury Press
Random House, 20 Vauxhall Bridge Road,
London SW1V 2SA

Random House Australia (Pty) Limited
20 Alfred Street, Milsons Point, Sydney,
New South Wales 2061, Australia

Random House New Zealand Limited
18 Poland Road, Glenfield,
Auckland 10, New Zealand

Random House South Africa (Pty) Limited
PO Box 337, Bergvlei, 2012 South Africa

Random House UK Limited Reg. No. 954009

A CIP catalogue record for this book
is available from the British Library

ISBN 0 09 933271 X

Designed by Roger Walker
Photography by Jon Stewart
Exercise clothing and trainers supplied by Nike

Printed and bound in Great Britain by
Cox & Wyman Ltd., Reading, Berkshire

CONTENTS

ACKNOWLEDGMENTS

With special thanks to:

Dr Penny Stanway for reading the manuscript so carefully and declaring Slim for Life medically sound;

Gail Pollard, SRD, Consultant Dietitian, also for reading the manuscript and checking the nutritional safety of the Eat to Slim system;

Tee Dobinson, AFFA Certification Specialist, for checking the safety of the exercise system in Step Five and for demonstrating the exercises;

All the people who kindly tested the Slim for Life system for me;

Tony Allen for much help in research and preparation of the manuscript;

Also, many thanks to Jan Bowmer, Jane Turnbull, Niccy Cowen, Anabel Briggs, Bob Hollingsworth, Roger Walker and all the team at Ebury.

WARNING

If you have a medical condition, or are pregnant, the diet and exercises described in this book should not be followed without first consulting your doctor. All guidelines and warnings should be read carefully and the author and publisher cannot accept responsibility for injuries or damage arising out of a failure to comply with the same.

INTRODUCTION

Have you spent years 'on' and 'off' diets, but are now actually heavier than you were to start with?

Have you lost weight successfully, only to put it all back on again?

Have you tried to slim and failed because you couldn't stand either the diet food or the deprivation?

Are you completely disillusioned with the whole idea of dieting, but still you *hate* being overweight?

If you answered 'yes' to one or more of those questions, then you are one of ten million people in this country who are fat and fed up – and this is the book for you.

Slim for Life will become your friend, your helper, your confidante, your tutor. It's a guidebook that will lead you to success because it doesn't just tell you to 'eat less': it helps you to see why you've been eating too much and shows you how to control your intake.

Slim for Life takes you, step by logical step, through a unique, new, exciting – and, yes, challenging – self-help programme which will ensure that you become slim and *stay* slim once and for all.

In *Slim for Life* there are no gimmicks; no promises about exactly how much weight you will lose in a given space of time. There is no 'set', tyrannical diet in this book, no forbidden foods, no dubious regimes to follow – and few, if any, rules. Yet you *will* lose weight if you work through the six-step programme at your own pace and don't progress to the next step until you have mastered the one before. And you will *keep* the weight off.

Because *Slim for Life* is a book to get you *thinking* and *doing* rather than just a book to read, and because there *is* so much in it for you to absorb and do, you may take not hours, or even days, but weeks to work through its pages. But when you consider the umpteen hours you have wasted trying and failing on previous diets, or simply on feeling miserable and despising your own body, it will be time you can afford.

It will also be time you enjoy – yes, I am confident that for the first time you will actually *enjoy* a book that is helping you to lose weight!

So what are the six steps that are the key to long-term slimness?

In **Step One**, you learn the importance of motivation – and find out your own particular strong motivators that will keep you slimming right down to the weight that is reasonable for you.

In **Step Two**, you will discover that it's *not* all your fault you're fat. I open your eyes to the real reasons you are overweight and take away the guilt you feel about your eating habits. Every person with a weight problem will find Step Two both a revelation and a great relief.

In **Step Three**, you learn how to control even the most wayward of eating habits. Whether your problem is yo-yo dieting, bingeing, a hefty appetite, addiction to a particular food, comfort eating, dislike of 'healthy' foods – or anything else – you will learn here how to take control. And by the end of this step you will probably already be losing weight.

In **Step Four**, you find out more about eating to slim and eating healthily without losing either taste or satisfaction. Here is where you build your own slimming programme to suit yourself. The system is totally flexible, works for anyone and is based on the easy-to-follow 'pyramid' style of eating.

In **Step Five**, you master the ways to overcome your resistance to using your body. I show you how to get moving and burn up extra calories without feeling bored, miserable, strained or martyred.

Then, in **Step Six**, you consolidate everything you have learnt, look to the future – and, I sincerely hope, help *me* to influence future generations, so that no one need ever go on a diet again!

So, now, if you want to be slim for life, turn the page and embark on an exciting journey that will end in long-term success. You don't need willpower: you just need some time and an open mind.

Together we can do it. Remember, if diets don't work for you, then this book will!

Check Out Your Motivation

You CAN do it – if you really want to!

How many times have you said: 'I haven't got the willpower to stick to a diet!'?

The truth is that neither 'willpower' nor, indeed, a traditional 'diet' are necessary in order for you to lose weight and keep it off. In fact 'willpower' – conjuring up pictures of heroic and tortuous self-denial, of ferocious battles against your bodily needs and signals – is the *last* thing you need.

You don't need willpower because you're never again going to be embarking on that sort of diet.

If the time is right for you to lose weight, and if you choose the right type of weight-loss plan for *you*, as far as slimming is concerned the word 'willpower' need never enter your vocabulary.

Everything you are going to learn in Steps Two, Three, Four, Five and Six will help you to understand why you have been eating and behaving in a way that has made you gain too much weight, and will teach you how to 'alter the balance' painlessly, so that losing weight, and keeping if off, becomes a natural and pleasurable process rather than a fight. And if there is no fight, there can be no loser, can there?

In Steps Two and Three – and beyond – you will be looking at yourself honestly, looking at your life honestly, and understanding yourself and your eating habits so that finally you can decide to be your own boss and at last control your weight, shape and wellbeing. What this will take is not willpower, but *motivation*.

All that motivation means, really, is wanting to be in shape more than you want to stay out of shape. It is strong self-motivation that leads to the *determination* to say: 'Yes, this time *I really do want to be slimmer – and I'm going to be.*'

The fact is that losing weight and shaping up, my way, *isn't* hard. It can be done. *You can do it*, once and for all. *Slim for Life* will show you how – if you let me. In fact, just by picking up *Slim for Life* and reading this far, you have taken a big step towards proving that, this time, you *do* have motivation. Together we can do the rest.

I say 'together' because this is a book you don't just sit and read through over the course of, say, a day. *Slim for Life,* all the way through, asks you to *do* things and if you use the book properly it will be a guide that is by your side for many weeks while you progress to the new, slimmer you.

One step at a time, you will think, discover, analyse, do, sort out problems, find out your best ways to lose weight. Together we work our way through to the end, ongoing result – a slimmer, fitter you for life.

Remember, the need and desire in you to achieve that result must be greater than the need or desire in you to continue as you are.

So let's get started on the programme now with your own personal MOTIVATION ASSESSMENT. For this you will just need a pen and some quiet time on your own so you can look into yourself and think about what in life *you* really want to be, do, give, and take.

YOUR MOTIVATION ASSESSMENT

In the following pages we will examine the eight major groups of motivating factors – the things that normally 'fire up people' most to get slimmer. These are appearance; short-term health; long-term health and longevity; wardrobe; sex and partnerships; career/work; everyday life; self-esteem/social relations.

These groups, I have found in my twenty years' experience of advising overweight people and talking to newly slim people and long-term ex-slimmers, comprise all the reasons that people set out to lose weight and to keep it off. Of course, your reasons may well be different from someone else's. What is important to you may mean nothing to the next person.

What I urge you to do is to read through all the section discussions and then, at the end of each one, you'll find a list of statements to tick whether you agree strongly, agree mildly, or disagree. You will notice, by the way, that I've started the statements with phrases such as 'I want ...' rather than 'I should ...' because feeling that you *should* do something is not a strong motivation. You must have a real want and need.

1. Appearance

No matter how many times we may hear feminists say that we should be proud and happy to be fat, or no matter how often radical writers try to tell us that it isn't 'politically correct' to take any notice of someone's size or appearance, the fact is that if we are not at, or near, a reasonable body weight for our frame, and reasonably in shape, we tend to feel unattractive. In Steps Two and Three we will be discussing in more detail the rights and wrongs of this feeling, but, for now, the important point is that for 99 per cent of us: if we look good, we feel good. And, for 99 per cent of us, looking good means looking slim and fit.

Don't feel guilty about wanting to lose weight because you long to look better. In survey after survey conducted amongst both men and women of all ages, the chief motive for wanting to lose weight is appearance.

I think one of the main reasons for this is that we live in a society where we frequently meet new people and where we have to sum others up – and be summed up ourselves – in seconds. All people have to go on at that first encounter is the way you look – and people will decide in an instant whether or not they want to talk to you, to be friends with you, or even, research shows, to employ you. Of course, it isn't just your size that has an impact – your expression, your tidiness, your body language, your choice of clothes, all these may figure – but if you are not happy with your size, this will, inevitably, be a part of what you project.

In other words, to make your mark all you have in so many life situations is the way you look *now*. Fair or unfair, it's true. Even if people aren't judging you that way you tend to feel that they are, and if you're aware that you don't look the best you could look your self-confidence is lowered.

The 'appearance motivation' factor may not be strong in you if you are pounds rather than stones overweight. Check out the statements on the facing page and judge for yourself.

2. Short-term health

Being overweight can affect your health in more ways than perhaps you realise.

Outlined here are some of the short-term health problems that obesity can cause or make worse. Even if you are not 'clinically obese' – i.e. 20 per cent or more over your reasonable weight – you may find that at least some of the problems apply to you.

Back pain Surplus weight – especially around the lower stomach area – coupled with weak stomach muscles, can place great strain on the lower back and is a major factor in low-back pain. Even a surplus stone (6.4 kg) can do this.

Varicose veins Excess weight causes unnecessary strain on the vascular system and, as your legs carry all your body weight, the result can be unsightly, and sometimes painful, varicose veins.

	Agree	*Slightly* *agree*	Disagree
● I want to look at myself in a mirror and feel pleased with what I see.	☐	☐	☐
● I want to feel happy enough with my looks to go swimming/wear a swimsuit /sit on the beach or [fill in your requirement]	☐	☐	☐
● I want to receive compliments on the way I look.	☐	☐	☐
● I want people to look at me and see me, a 'normal-weight person', not an 'overweight person'.	☐	☐	☐
● I want my appearance to reflect the person I am – which is not fat.	☐	☐	☐
● I want to live the rest of my life in a body I can feel proud of.	☐	☐	☐
● I want [fill in any other statement of your choosing]	☐	☐	☐

Number of *Agrees* ☐   Number of *Slightly agrees* ☐

Shortness of breath   If you are overweight your lungs have to work harder to supply your body volume with oxygen. This is one reason why the risk while under anaesthetic is greater for fat people. Excess weight also places more strain on your heart and is thereby a contributing factor in the increased incidence of heart disease amongst overweight people. In the short term, an increased tendency to breathlessness may be an indication that your lungs and heart are not coping well with your weight.

Infertility   Statistics show that if you want a baby your chances of becoming pregnant are diminished if you are obese.

Pregnancy problems   Being overweight during pregnancy can lead to raised blood pressure and the increased possibility of complications. Childbirth, too, can be more difficult if you are obese.

Skin complaints   Overweight people often complain of sore rough skin and rashes caused either through increased perspiration or skin surfaces rubbing together (e.g. on the inside thighs).

	Agree	Slightly agree	Disagree
• I prefer to live inside a body that is as healthy as I can make it.	☐	☐	☐
• At least part of my state of health is something over which I have control.	☐	☐	☐
• It would give me peace of mind to think that I am not in any way abusing my body through what I eat or drink.	☐	☐	☐

Number of *Agrees* ☐   Number of *Slightly agrees* ☐

3. Long-term health

As time goes on, most of us who are perhaps just moderately overweight become more overweight. And, as time goes on, the possibility of increased weight affecting our health becomes greater and even more worrying. The more overweight you are, and the longer you have been overweight (the two usually go hand in hand), the greater is the likelihood that you have developed, or will develop, one or more of the following:

Immobility to some degree – obese people tend to move more slowly and less often than slim people and to be reluctant to take part in activities – leading to long-term lack of fitness.

Hypertension (high blood pressure)   People with high blood pressure are more likely to suffer from both stroke and heart disease.

Atherosclerosis   This is the narrowing of the arteries by fatty deposits which restricts the flow of blood and leads to a greater risk of a stroke or heart attack. Latest research shows that even if arterial narrowing has already occurred, in many patients this can be reversed with a low-fat diet.

Gallstones   The majority of people who develop gallstones are female and the majority of these are overweight females.

Osteoarthritis   Overweight people are more likely to develop osteoarthritis (except, surprisingly, of the hip). Once this is present, their excess weight places more strain and more pain on the weight-bearing knee joints.

Mid-life onset diabetes   The type of diabetes that begins in or around middle age is much more likely to occur if you are overweight. Reducing your weight if you have this form of diabetes can often completely control the condition without drugs.

Some forms of cancer   Obese males have a higher incidence of colon, rectum and prostate cancer; females of gallbladder, breast, ovary and uterus cancers.

Obviously, then, obesity has the very real capacity to diminish the quality of your life by undermining your health and it may also contribute to a shortening of your potential lifespan.

	Agree	Slightly agree	Disagree
• I want to do everything I can to prevent unnecessary health problems in later life.	☐	☐	☐
• I would like to lose weight to help my [fill in your complaint here]	☐	☐	☐
• I want to live to a healthy old age and be active enough to enjoy playing with my grand-children or [you say what]	☐	☐	☐
• It will be easier for me to tackle a weight problem now than to wait until the problem is larger and more of a health problem.	☐	☐	☐

Number of *Agrees* ☐   Number of *Slightly agrees* ☐

4. Wardrobe

There is little in life more demoralising – and, indeed, annoying – than having a wardrobe of perfectly good clothes that you can't wear because they don't fit you any longer. This is one of the main motivators for people without a great deal of weight to lose. I know to my own cost that when I was 10 lbs (4.5 kg) overweight (mostly around my middle) I couldn't get into any of my trousers, jeans or skirts.

Neither is there anything much more depressing than wanting something new to wear but feeling dread at the thought of going near a clothes shop because you know that (a) not much will fit you, (b) not much that does fit you will look good on you, and (c) what, if anything, you end up with will probably not be what you'd buy if you were slimmer. And even if what you wear doesn't figure high on your list of priorities *before* you lose weight, I have found that almost everyone who does slim – a little or a lot – is absolutely delighted at how much easier 'wardrobe management' becomes and realises how much pleasure from feeling good in his or her clothes has been lacking in the past.

	Agree	Slightly agree	Disagree
• I want to be able to get back into all those clothes in my wardrobe.	☐	☐	☐
• I want to be able to go and choose some new clothes without being restricted by my size.	☐	☐	☐
• I want to look nice in fitted clothes.	☐	☐	☐
• I want to look nice in [fill in – e.g., jeans]	☐	☐	☐
• I want to feel relaxed in a changing-room.	☐	☐	☐

Number of *Agrees* ☐   Number of *Slightly agrees* ☐

5. Sex and partnerships

Your size shouldn't affect your enjoyment of sex or your attraction for the opposite sex, but all too often it does. This usually has as much to do with your lack of confidence with a partner when you feel unattractive as it has to do with the fact that most people do prefer a partner to be a reasonable body weight. Once a prospective partner gets to know you he or she may well not mind what size you are, but, sadly, too many relationships that could be good never get started because of that initial prejudice.

7. *Everyday life*

One woman who used to be 15 stone (95.3 kg) and is now 10 stone (63.5 kg) wrote to me explaining what it was that finally made her lose her surplus weight. It was when she admitted to herself that the reason she had always refused to enter the mother's race at her son's school sports day was not that she didn't like losing (the reason she'd always given him) but that she couldn't bear the thought of being stared at as she ran. She was ashamed of her bulk. 'I'd spent years trying to slim but it was that one thing that spurred me on.' The next year, having lost weight and become fitter, she took part in the race and came third. Not only was she slimmer, she'd proved to herself she didn't *have* to lose, either! She has also realised how, through being fat, she missed so many of the pleasures of parenthood – unable to go on bike rides, to give piggyback rides, or even to share a bath because there wasn't room!

Everyone who loses a lot of weight says that day-to-day life is so much more pleasant, and easier, when you're not carrying around loads of heavy surplus baggage. And being slimmer opens up so many more life possibilities.

If your weight problem amounts to only a stone (6.4 kg) or so, you may not find that your life is restricted in this way; but, remember, weight usually creeps on and eventually this could be your problem too. Check out the statements on the facing page.

8. *Self-esteem/social relations*

Many of the motivating factors we have already looked at are linked in some way with your own self-esteem and the boost it gets when you lose weight. But your surplus weight and the almost inevitable drop in self-esteem it brings are a lethal combination with regard to your social life and social interaction.

Even after so many years of professional involvement with people of all shapes and sizes, I continue to be amazed at how drastically our size affects what we do and how we behave with others – friends, strangers, family, neighbours.

	Agree	Slightly agree	Disagree
• I want to be able to live my life without having my size affect what I do.	☐	☐	☐
• I want to live my life without being almost permanently conscious of my weight.	☐	☐	☐
• I want to be able to run a few metres without getting breathless.	☐	☐	☐
• I want to be able easily to tie my shoelaces and put on tights/socks.	☐	☐	☐
• I want to be able to play active games with the kids.	☐	☐	☐
• I want to be able to sit in seats on public transport without a squeeze.	☐	☐	☐
• I want to feel cool in hot weather, not hot and bothered.	☐	☐	☐
• I want to get through a busy day without aching legs and feet at the end.	☐	☐	☐
• I want to get through a busy day without feeling physically exhausted.	☐	☐	☐
• I want to enjoy having my photo taken.	☐	☐	☐
• [Fill in your lifestyle desire]	☐	☐	☐

Number of *Agrees* ☐   Number of *Slightly agrees* ☐

Very often it is of course a lack of self-esteem and self-confidence that leads you to overeat in the first place; the excess weight then simply reinforces your low opinion of yourself. If this is the case, you have to work on the original problems that made you fat, as well as on your weight (which we'll be doing in Steps Two and Three). But it has been proved time and again that when people lose unrequired weight they gain the confidence and the spark to deal more effectively with all kinds of people.

So, whether your overweight condition is turning you into a lonely stay-at-home, you're everyone's favourite agony aunt but would rather not be, or you are the life and soul of the party who secretly longs to be something else, check this list.

	Agree	Slightly agree	Disagree
• I'd love to go out more than I do but I've lost my confidence.	☐	☐	☐
• I would love to meet new people without feeling inferior.	☐	☐	☐
• I wish I could feel as confident 'in person' as I do on the telephone.	☐	☐	☐
• I don't initiate friendships because I feel people will be put off because of my size. I would like to change this.	☐	☐	☐
• I feel I often behave like a 'fat person' when I really want to be *me*.	☐	☐	☐
• I am sure that being overweight has isolated me.	☐	☐	☐
• I can't relax socially because I feel awkward about my size.	☐	☐	☐

(continued)	Agree	Slightly agree	Disagree
• I am thoroughly fed up with my size dictating my social life!	☐	☐	☐
• I pretend to be 'fat and happy' but really I'm not.	☐	☐	☐
• I am sure that being overweight has altered my natural personality. I'm			
— more aggressive	☐	☐	☐
— more shy	☐	☐	☐
— more pliable	☐	☐	☐
— [or fill in differently]	☐	☐	☐
• I deliberately avoid situations where I'll meet new people because I can't bear them thinking of me as a 'fat person'.	☐	☐	☐

Number of *Agrees* ☐   Number of *Slightly agrees* ☐

HOW DID YOU GET ON?

Whether you agreed with just a few of the statements or with most of them, I bet that at this moment you are picturing yourself slim and imagining how much better your life will be then. That is marvellous – it means you are focusing now on what you want, and, until you do that, you can't *achieve* what you want.

You may have found that what you consider to be your main motivator wasn't listed. In that case it is likely to be one of the following:

A short-term motivator, such as 'I want to slim for my wedding' or 'I want to slim for my holiday'. The motivators included on the previous pages are more general hopes and ideas, concerning ongoing things rather than short-term goals. This is deliberate because, if you are really going to lose your weight and keep it off for good, you need something more than a short-term goal. Okay, so you lose your weight for a wedding or a holiday – then, when that event is over, you put it all back on again. Little goals along the way, such as losing a few pounds in time for a specific date, may be of help to some people but they shouldn't be your sole reason for slimming. They tend to encourage 'yo-yo' dieting, which we are trying to avoid.

A negative motivator. Any motivator that begins with the opening words 'I should' or 'I must' (.... 'lose weight because I know I need to) is not likely to be incentive enough. Also, any motivator that comes from someone else (e.g. 'My doctor says I should lose weight for my health') is a poor motivator. Lastly, any motivator born out of fear or panic (e.g. 'I am going to slim because my husband says he will leave me if I don't') isn't likely to succeed, either. If you are slimming for other people, it may work for a while, but not long-term. And in cases where you are slimming out of duty or fear, you build up resentment and other negative emotions and won't be able to keep it up. *You slim for you*.

An impossible expectation. Losing weight can definitely improve your life in many ways, but don't, please, kid yourself that losing weight will be the answer to all your problems. Slim people have problems, too. So if you thought your motivator was, say, 'I want to lose half a stone (3.2 kg) because I know it will make my husband love me more', or 'I want to lose weight so I will look just like Julia Roberts [or whoever]', then I can't agree with you. The gain or loss of 7 lbs (3.2 kg) never made someone stop loving you or start loving you. And if you lose weight you will look like yourself, only slimmer. You can't expect perfection because there is no such thing. Even the people you *think* are perfect aren't. And to embark on a slimming campaign in the hope that you will end up that way is to invite failure – because you will end up dissatisfied.

Don't expect miracles from weight loss. Instead, be motivated by objectives that are achievable. That way you will succeed, not only now, but for life.

Go through the motivator lists again and note which sections seemed to involve you most. Practise focusing on the things you want to achieve. Transfer to a sheet of paper those motivators you consider to be the most important – say, the top ten (or, if you didn't have that many, write out in order of importance the ones you did have).

Refer to this list frequently throughout your slimming campaign and, especially, at the end of every Step in this book. Keep it in your wallet or purse or whatever you carry round with you most of the time. *Do this* right away. I will come back to this list later.

Now you've written out your list, how do you feel? Optimistic that at last you really are going to do it? Keen to begin? Positive and strong? I hope you feel all those, but perhaps too there's a niggling little doubt somewhere at the back of your mind? A feeling a bit like when you were at school and about to take an exam you really wanted to pass and really knew you could pass, but, nevertheless, you still couldn't convince yourself you'd done enough revision? You may be feeling 'yes, the time *is* right to slim now, but am I really up to the task ahead?'

Here are some of the things that may be at the back of your mind. We might as well get them out into the open.

Doubts such as:
- However clever or experienced in slimming the author of this book is, can she really get my weight off? Wasn't I just 'born to be fat'?
- I've failed on so many diets; why should I win this time just because I want to?

- How on earth can I lose weight without cutting out all the things I like best?

Fears such as:
- I'm frightened of feeling hungry.
- I'm frightened of failing.

Practicalities such as:
- However much I want to lose weight, how can I do it on my income?
- How can I possibly keep to a slimming diet when all my family eat like horses?

Guilt such as:
- Should I really be spending all this time and effort on myself when there are so many other demands on my time?

Yes, you *are* feeling things of this sort? Well, don't worry. That is fine. It is normal and it means you are not being unrealistic and burying your head in the sand about possible problems that may lie ahead.

What every overweight person needs to do before he or she can slim successfully is to examine closely these feelings and problems and find ways of dealing with each and every one of them. There is nothing that worries you now that we can't deal with effectively. We can replace or redefine all negatives and problems with positives and solutions.

In Steps Two and Three we are going to take a new look at food and at your eating habits and I'm going to show you that you *do* have the determination, the capacity and the ability to slim and stay slim for life. Don't be impatient. Don't think I'm trying to hold you back. After all, if you've been struggling for years with excess weight and failing to lose it, what's your hurry? Think of all the time you've wasted – now you're going to use it wisely. And, anyway, even if you don't realise it, your slimming campaign has already begun. It started the minute you opened this book. We're already doing it. You're already on your way to slimness.

YOU CAN DO IT!

Yes, you *can* do it! Try this exercise now to prove to yourself that you can focus on a target.

All you have to do is choose one thing to do each day for the following week – something that you normally fight shy of doing. It can be anything at all as long as it isn't connected with food, isn't unpleasant and will help you feel good and positive if you do it.

Here are some of my suggestions. You can use any of these or make up your own list, then pick one for each day.

My list

- Smile and say 'good-morning' to people you pass in the street.
- Ring up someone you haven't spoken to for a long time and have been worrying that you'll lose touch with altogether.
- Clean the oven (or similar chore).
- Voice your point of view in a discussion when normally you'd stay silent.
- Pay someone you like a compliment or tell them you like them.
- Go and introduce yourself to new neighbours down the road.
- Be pleasant all day to someone at work with whom you've never got on particularly well before.

Your list

- ....
- ....
- ....
- ....
- ....
- ....
- ....

Well, how did you get on? Even if you didn't manage to do all seven, congratulate yourself for doing what you did. How did you feel? It is not always easy to do things you are not in the habit of doing, even if they are pleasant things or little things. But when you see you have the power to make life a little bit nicer – both for yourself and for other people – you'll find yourself gaining confidence to do more, to be more outgoing. You can actually train yourself to adopt new, more positive ways of behaviour.

What reaction did you get to the things you did that involved other people? Say, you phoned an old friend you were in danger of losing touch with. I bet that friend was delighted, not grumpy – and I bet *you* felt much better afterwards, too!

What you will have discovered by trying out this small exercise is that taking control is much more pleasing, satisfying – and fun – than being passive.

Now try another exercise. Make a list below of all the things, big and little, that you have done/can do well in your life. Don't say 'nothing'; think about it. Here are some suggestions of the kind of things I mean:

- I won a school prize for writing.
- I scored a winning double in the darts team.
- I'm good at cutting hair.
- I can sing.
- I can drive a car.
- I can ride a horse.
- I can use a computer.

Your list

- ....
- ....
- ....
- ....
- ....
- ....
- ....

I expect you've filled that space up and need more room, so use some paper of your own. Go on, keep thinking and write everything down!

Now, if you can do, or did do, *all that* – whether it is now or was ten years ago – you can lose your extra weight and keep it off.

STEP ONE ROUND-UP

Go back and read your top ten motivators again. Now read this list of statements and tick the ones you agree with:

- ☐ I feel more positive than negative.
- ☐ I wasn't 'born to be fat'.
- ☐ I am willing to take a close and honest look at myself and at what influences my eating habits.
- ☐ I want to be slim for life.
- ☐ I can be slim for life.

If you ticked all of the above statements, you are now ready to move on to Step Two. Step Two will be a fascinating journey for you. It is where you will find out about the 'shape saboteurs' – the factors that have been contriving to keep you overweight and undermining all your best intentions. Believe me, it's *not* all your fault you're fat!

Get Wise to the Shape Saboteurs

It's NOT all your fault you're fat!

I can tell you straight away *what* has made you overweight. You are overweight because you have been taking in too many calories (probably fatty and/or sugary calories) for your body's needs. That is a simple fact. However, *why* you have done this is a different, less simple matter.

Why we are overweight and why we fail to stick to diets has, usually, little to do with greed, weak will, and so forth, but a lot to do with outside influences. It is all these outside influences that I have called the 'shape saboteurs' and here, in Step Two, we are going to learn all about these saboteurs and how they have been keeping you fat, making you fatter, or stopping you from losing weight. The saboteurs are many and varied; you'll probably have been totally unaware of at least some of them. But the truth is that we live in a society geared towards encouraging us to overeat; then, when we do, it makes us feel guilty about it and suddenly the problem is all ours!

Well, *not any longer*. You can stop feeling guilty about your size – and about any past failures to lose weight – *right now*. You are about to find out that what you have probably been calling your 'excuses' are, in fact, perfectly valid reasons for having a weight problem in the first place and also for not having been able to do much about it *so far*. This doesn't mean that if there have been valid reasons for your weight problem it is therefore useless you ever thinking that you can get slim. Far from it. When you fully understand – as you soon will – what has been keeping you fat, then, and only then, will you be able to do something about it once and for all; then, and only then, will it finally be your choice if you decide not to act on your new knowledge but to stay out of shape.

Since it is not all your fault, I don't ask you to take the blame for your size. But what I will, in Step Three, ask you to do is to take *responsibility* for doing something about it. And be assured that the solutions are not difficult: they may take time and they make take practice, but they're *not* hard.

You *can* be slim for life! But, first, let's find out just who or what those shape saboteurs really are....

WHO ARE THE SHAPE SABOTEURS?

The rest of Step Two is divided into four sections, each of which deals with a particular aspect of shape sabotage. These are:

1. Food, glorious food – a close look at how our basic instincts, food availability and its promotion all make us overeat.

2. Circumstances 'beyond my control'? – a discussion of the lifestyle and personal factors that you may feel are stopping you from being slim.

3. The VIPs – a look through the microscope at the Very Interested People around you. Do your friends, family and colleagues really have your best interests at heart?

4. The 'tyrannical' diet – an explanation, especially for failed ex-dieters, as to how and when a diet can produce negative results.

Each section will probably apply to you, to a greater or lesser degree, and I'd like you to read the whole of Step Two thoroughly even if one or more sections doesn't seem particularly relevant to you. But to help you decide straight away which of the shape saboteurs has had the most influence on you, at the start of each of the four sections you will find a list of statements relating to food and eating, with boxes alongside them to tick.

Read through these statements and tick whichever ones you agree with. The more you tick in a section, the more influence that section is likely to have had, or to be having, on your eating patterns. Each of the four sections relates directly and in sequence to the four sections in Step Three, where we learn how to beat the shape saboteurs and get slim. So if, for instance, you have a lot of statements ticked here in, say, sections 2 and 4, you will know that it will be particularly important for you to do extra work on sections 2 and 4 in Step Three.

SECTION 1:

Food, Glorious Food!

The scandal of our national diet

Tick which statements apply to you

☐ I don't really eat much, yet I'm fat.

☐ However much I cut down on food, I can't lose weight.

☐ I like fatty foods and all the 'wrong' foods.

☐ I can resist certain fatty foods but am addicted to one or two.

☐ I don't enjoy 'healthy' foods so how can I diet?

☐ I've always had a sweet tooth.

☐ When I see food and it's available, I eat it even if I'm not hungry.

☐ If I open a pack of something, I can't stop eating until it's empty.

☐ I always eat up everything I'm given.

☐ I'm not a comfort eater, I just really enjoy my food.

☐ I've got a big appetite.

☐ I can't bear the idea of feeling hungry.

☐ Food is one of my few pleasures in life.

☐ I love to eat and drink with friends.

If you ticked several of the above statements, you're one of millions of victims of a Western society that has, over the past forty years, created an ever-widening gap between our food intake and our energy output. In other words, as a nation we are eating more (especially of the wrong types of fatty, sugary foods) and taking less exercise than ever before.

Where once, for thousands of years, without even thinking about it, man managed to balance what he ate with how much energy he used, now modern life has made that seemingly simple equation hard to achieve for many of us ... so we get fat. With a third or more of men and women in this country overweight, and approximately 10 per cent clinically obese (i.e. *very* overweight), it is a collective national problem and in the long term needs to be dealt with in that way.

To see what has gone wrong, we need to go right back to the Stone Age. Early man lived by hunting and gathering what he could find. Without the means of storage and not knowing when he would eat again, he would consume everything that was available. Occasionally this meant that he would have a feast and perhaps lay down fat stores in his body. But at other times food would be hard to find and he would have to use that fat for energy, so he would get slim again. At that time food was plain, unadulterated meat or fish and wholefoods – nuts, berries, leaves and so on. No wonder no Stone Age man or woman had to worry about his or her waistline!

But, as humans progressed over the centuries towards today's society, things began to change – at first, slowly; then, in the last few decades, with speed.

By as long ago as the sixteenth century, the more wealthy Europeans were suffering from obesity. In fact, until the mid 1800s fatness was often seen as a sign of affluence and was therefore something to be admired: you were sufficiently well off to be able to afford to eat plenty. Sugar, for instance, cost in the sixteenth century the equivalent of what caviare costs today.

Through the centuries, agriculture and food production, transport, storage and preservation methods improved considerably and so, by the mid 1800s, obesity was no longer the province of the rich, as for many people more food was available than they actually needed. But they still ate it – as we do today – with one corner of the mind unchanged since Stone Age times and fearing, perhaps, that *next* week they may not have *anything*.

During this period, dieting to lose weight began to be a topic of major conversation – and, about that time, Messrs Fry and Cadbury discovered how to make chocolate!

But it wasn't until the mid twentieth century that the British girth began to expand in earnest. Here's what happened:

We had World War II   During the war, food rationing was introduced and, afterwards, when asked what two commodities they had missed most, Britons answered: 'Sugar and butter.' After the (literally) lean times of the war, when rationing of those products ended, we could hardly wait to indulge ourselves. Mums began to experiment with rich dishes in the kitchen – and, as it now seemed almost criminal to waste any form of food, children everywhere were made to 'eat everything up' and never leave a scrap. There was real pleasure in seeing families able to eat their fill.

We grew more sophisticated   With safe air travel and more money to spend, we began holidaying abroad. This made us aware that there was a whole world of wonderful tastes and new and exciting foods out there. The American influence became stronger: suddenly we all wanted fridges and freezers, and hamburgers and chips. In research experiments it has been proved that we eat much more when we have a wide variety of foods to choose from rather than just a few.

By the 1960s, most of us had televisions, too – at which point the food manufacturers began to realise the huge power of advertising their wares on our screens.

We began eating out more   The '70s saw a huge growth in restaurants, cafés, pubs, fast food, wine bars and takeaway eating, matching our modern cosmopolitan lives. We also became accustomed to eating in each other's homes as a matter of course. And 'novel' meals that we haven't had to prepare ourselves always invite us to eat more.

We were offered convenience foods to match our busy lifestyles The pace of life in the '60s, '70s and '80s seemed to get faster and faster for all age groups, young and old, male and female. And eventually everything we wanted for the table could be bought ready prepared and ready to eat. Any time we were hungry we no longer had to clean, prepare, cook and wait; we could have it instantly. With the advent of the microwave oven, our instant-eating programme was complete. Now we could – and often did – eat four times as much in a quarter of the time it would have taken in the '50s.

We were offered convenience gadgets and cars Whereas once we walked or cycled to work – or, indeed, spent most of our day at home being active – now we bought cars or train tickets to get us to work and would spend our days off going for a spin in the car instead of taking a bike ride. At the same time there was available a positive forest of 'labour-saving' equipment which reduced to a minimum the amount of time we spent on housework, gardening, car cleaning and food preparation. And watching television suddenly seemed much more appealing than actually *doing* anything, so that our new physical inactivity was compounded: evenings were spent sitting in squashy chairs, watching TV – and eating!

But isn't this all of our own choosing?
No! We have been nudged in subtle and not so subtle ways along paths not quite of our own choice. And, of course, the collective trend of society is hard to move against unless the individual realises what is happening.

So if you think you always choose the food you eat, think again. Someone else is giving you a helping hand.

Offers you can't refuse   Our food industry is a powerful, lobbying force which, overall, makes huge profits, even in times of recession. One of the reasons for this is that it is practised at capitalising on all our deepest survival instincts. Its most successful companies know that we still have an inclination to eat when food is there – because tomorrow it may not be. They recognise that it is instinctive to eat food or want food when we see it. They know that it is natural to stock up for possible hard times ahead. And they also know that, as breast milk is sweet and fatty, we have an inborn liking for sweet, fatty foods – one that should fade as we outgrow the breast, but that is easy to nurture and turn into a lifelong addiction.

You need only take a look at one or two issues of the grocery trade's 'bible', *The Grocer* magazine, to realise too that the food industry is well aware that the more 'added value' products it can sell to us, the more profit there is to be made.

Put simply, there is more money to be made selling a cream cake than there is in selling a carrot. The carrot is a natural product that just needs to be grown, dug up, perhaps washed and sorted, and transported to the shop. But the cake has gone through a manufacturing process which has turned often basically cheap ingredients such as sugar and fat into a relatively expensive product.

And, by producing and promoting 'added value' lines, the manufacturers can capitalise on another of our latent instincts – the enthusiasm for 'novel' foods. If the customer's palate becomes a little jaded with one particular kind of fatty, sugary cake, the manufacturer will alter an ingredient, call it something 'new' – and there you are, back eating it again.

If we all ate nothing but natural items that hadn't gone through several processes before they arrive in the shops, we would all eat far less – and the British food industry would collapse almost instantly. Not surprisingly, therefore, we are persuaded in various ways and by various means to continue buying the foods that make most profit.

Here are some of the ways you end up eating more than you might have done if you were left to your own devices:

Self-service: tempting you to buy more   The old-style local grocery shops that largely disappeared when the big supermarkets took off were not designed to get you to buy more food. You went along (probably with a short list) and you asked for what you wanted. Comparatively little food was on display and therefore you were generally not tempted into impulse buying through spotting something you just *had* to have. And, as you would probably be walking home, you'd be disinclined to buy too much since it would be too heavy or awkward to carry.

Nowadays, you go to the supermarket – and, if you still have a corner shop, it may have turned self-service too. Usually you get there by car so you can buy as much as you can put in the boot. You collect a big trolley, even if you only intend to buy a few goods. The first thing that hits you is probably the aroma of bread baking (which in many cases is piped through to the entrance from the in-store bakery). Just feel your appetite rising!

Even if you have a shopping list, as you push your trolley around, you find yourself putting in more and more extra goods. Taste testings, special multi-buy offers, money-off packs, tempting visual displays – and the very need to walk past things you hadn't intended to buy in order to get to what you did want – all encourage you. Add to that your increasing hunger and then the wait at the checkout, where often you find a display of confectionery, and there you are, buying chocolate bars too!

And who *doesn't* sell food these days?   Even if you don't visit the supermarket and don't have any intention of buying food, food is around almost everywhere, begging you to buy it. Go for some petrol, walk to the desk to pay – and there is the confectionery. Go to buy a paper – and there are the packet snacks and the chocolate bars. Go to the garden centre, even, and you'll find anything from a pick-and-mix display of sweets to preserves and biscuits next to the houseplants. Vending machines are everywhere; so are takeout shops, mini sandwich bars and street food stalls.

And one thing is for sure: not one of them is selling carrots. They are all selling *fat* and *sugar*.

The power of advertising   Once you get home and switch on the TV or open a magazine, the real persuasion to buy begins. Advertising is what really drives you towards those food and drink products that otherwise you might not have bought.

And, again, it is not carrots (or, generally, any fresh fruit or vegetable) that are being advertised. It is value-added lines. As I write, the latest list of the Top 20 foods advertised on TV is composed almost entirely of fatty, sugary and 'snack' products. In one year, the food companies spent more money on advertising these Top 20 foods than we as a nation spent on buying one staple 'healthy' natural product. The sum £175,200,000 was spent on TV advertising of the twenty foods, while just £100,800,000 was spent on buying long-grain rice in 1992!

The list of twenty foods didn't include confectionery. Over £95 *million* a year goes on advertising chocolate and sweets, a sum that is obviously well worth it as no less than £4,000,000,000 worth of confectionery was sold in 1992.

The reason these megasums are spent on TV advertising is that it works. When a product is advertised, its sales go up. Retailers are also more likely to stock a new product, or will stock more of an old favourite, if they know it is being advertised on TV or in the media.

The low-fat con   Let's be fair. The food industry has developed a whole array of low- or lower-fat products, such as skimmed milk, low-fat yogurt, low-fat spread and reduced-fat cheese, to meet a growing demand for 'healthier' produce from the public. And sales of these reduced-fat items (and other reduced-sugar ones) are growing all the time.

But there is an interesting twist to this. Yes, we are buying more of the reduced-fat items. But, overall, our national fat intake *hasn't* decreased in the past decade.

What is happening is that as fast as we swop to skimmed milk, etc. we are replacing that missing fat in our diets with more 'treat' items, such as luxury desserts, chocolate and pastries. So while fat and sugar are being removed from one set of products, they are, in effect, being put back into us via another set! For instance, just as we get into the habit of buying low-fat yogurt, we find we can now buy thick, whole-milk yogurts with added cream. Sales of those, and of new luxury ice-cream brands, are rising every week.

Bigger is better?   Despite the current economic recession, ours is a reasonably affluent society and we buy more food of all kinds – not just fat and sugar – than we used to. We are encouraged in this practice not only by all the ways I've described, but also by the manufacturers providing bigger pack sizes of old favourites, more items per multipack, more weight per instant meal – extra 25 per cent free – and so on. Everything, it sometimes seems, always has to be bigger to be better ... and to sell more.

This translates to bigger portions on our plates and in our mouths. Hunger is nothing but a distant memory, satiety a permanent feeling.

The fact is, because food is there and all around us in ever vaster amounts, and sold to us so very well, we eat it. We don't think about it: we just buy it and eat it. It is fashionable for feminists and psychologists to label those who have a weight problem as 'compulsive eaters'. Somehow we are made to feel that eating is always linked with psychological disorders, anti-feminism, oppression, depression, and so on. That may be part of the story, but I believe that the main reason we eat unwisely is that it is what our society has spent forty years or more persuading us to do.

We have been conditioned and encouraged, by a profit-motivated industry and a government largely funded by that industry itself, to eat a national diet that has made us fat.

Ironically, the Government has only recently realised what a serious national health problem obesity is, and is now at last trying to do something about it. In its White Paper (July 1992) *The Health of the Nation*, it set out targets for reducing the nation's fat-intake and obesity. It pledges to step up research into the factors that influence our choice of foods and aims to persuade manufacturers to produce more low-fat, low-sugar items, while the Government itself seeks better ways to get across the message that a high-fat diet can kill.

This is not before time – and in Step Six we'll be looking at more ways *you* can influence what we eat in Britain today and in the future.

It is natural to enjoy food and eating – you have to enjoy what you eat to survive. Don't feel guilty about taking pleasure in your meals. That doesn't need to change.

What is not natural is a diet so high in the types of food you have been so cleverly convinced that you do enjoy – the obesity-producing foods that make you crave more, more, more ....

What is not natural is eating a high-fat diet without having to hunt for it.

What is not natural is eating food when you aren't hungry and when you know that there isn't a scarcity round the corner.

Early man knew what we have been persuaded to forget: that food is a fuel to keep your body healthy, and should be enjoyed as such.

The good news is that once you have understood the hidden social and commercial factors that have been at work inducing you to eat more than you need, and encouraging you to develop ever-greater cravings for sweet and fatty foods, it is not too difficult to decide to take your own path. The right choices and foods are there, available to all of us.

In Step Three, I am going to show you how to continue enjoying food, glorious food by eating it in a slightly altered balance so that it becomes less fattening and more healthy.

I am going to show you how to make the supermarkets your friend and how to distinguish between appetite and hunger; how to eat only when *you* really want to and how to bring to the surface long-buried responses and instincts so that you – and not the food-pushers – control what goes into your mouth.

SECTION 2:

Circumstances 'Beyond My Control'?

'With my problems, how can I diet?'

Tick which statements apply to you

☐ I lead such a busy life that there's no time to think about myself.

☐ I feel guilty if I spend time on myself when there's so much to do for my family/boss/business/friends.

☐ Every day I intend to pay attention to myself and my diet but the day goes so quickly and at the end I've done nothing.

☐ With the life I lead I have to grab what food and drink I can.

☐ I haven't got the money to diet.

☐ I'm totally reliant on other people to feed me.

☐ I work shiftwork, so organising a slimming diet is impossible.

☐ I spend my life around food – shopping, preparing, cooking, clearing up. It's no wonder I'm fat.

☐ I'm tied to the house all day, I turn to food for comfort.

☐ I haven't got any friends around here and I feel lonely. Food cheers me up.

☐ I'm so depressed since I split with my partner. I find eating is some consolation.

☐ With my monthly PMS how can I control what I eat?

☐ I haven't been able to control my weight since I reached menopause.

☐ I've got a slow metabolism.

If you ticked many of the above statements, the life that you've chosen – or that has chosen you – appears to be conspiring to keep you overweight. Or, in the case of the last three statements, it's your hormones that are conspiring against you!

These are the kind of problems that people who aren't overweight will dismiss as excuses. They are not. They are, on the surface, valid reasons why you have had trouble losing weight and/or keeping it off.

And, again, modern society has a lot to answer for. So much has changed over the past fifty years or so in the way we live. We all expect to put a lot more into life and to get a lot more out of it. This means that if we *do* get that, we're busy, rushed, pressurised and stressed – and one of the ways we deal with that is by eating. If we *don't* get it – if, somehow, life seems to pass us by, and we're lonely, bored, out of work, miserable, restricted, we get stressed by that, too – and one of the ways we deal with that is by eating.

These are all 'lifestyle factors' that often make us feel we are swimming against the tide. Whether you're a superwoman trying to juggle kids, home, career and relationships; whether you're a college-leaver stuck at home because you can't find a job; or whether you're a single parent – whatever your situation, how you eat and what you eat is tightly bound up with that lifestyle.

I believe that our lifestyles have changed so much over the past fifty years or so that we haven't really come to terms with the changes.

The shifting population Before transport became so quick and easy, communications so good and organisations more global, people tended to stay in, or near, the area where they were born, where family, long-term friends and long-term associations all fostered a feeling of belonging. Today that lifestyle belongs to just a few. Today many of us live miles away from childhood friends, parents, grandparents, uncles and aunts. When we grow up, we leave home and then when our children grow up, so do they. We're fragmented and increasingly isolated. Even husbands and wives are often parted by long-distance commuting and work pressures. Divorce rates are high and separation increases the isolation even further. Now 25 per cent of homes are under single occupancy and we can feel just as isolated in the middle of a city as in a country cottage. Finally, for many people unemployment has been the last straw, when they have been denied the opportunity to find friendship with colleagues at work or enough money to socialise.

The shifting population, restlessly in search of jobs, better jobs, more desirable environments and greater prestige, has led to the break-up of the family unit – and food has replaced family and roots as our security, our comfort.

Having it all For women, the last two or three decades have brought sweeping changes in expectations – in what is expected of them and in what they expect of themselves. Filling in time with a 'little job' before finding a husband, having children and becoming a fully supported housewife, a sequence of events that was once the norm for many women, now sounds like the most ludicrous, old-fashioned custom ever. Though there has been a small return to the idea that it isn't such a terribly boring thing to want to stay at home and bring up the kids, women who do this almost always feel guilty or inferior. But the ones who do try to have it all – job, career, partner, kids and stylish home – and who also try to be fabulous cook, carer, fashion plate and do-it-yourself person all at once, feel guilty too, even

if they don't admit it and, either way, the body suffers. Housewives and most unemployed women and men stay at home ....
and eat. Busy 'juggling' women generally pay no attention to
their food intake ... and may end up eating too much by default.

'New man' – the vanishing species   And, of course, the whole
concept of 'having it all' has subtly changed. Women should
admit that what they really have is a situation that could be called
'*doing* it all'. Not only have they taken on half of the chores that
men used to feel *they* had to do – the gardening, do-it-yourself,
washing the car – but women are also still doing all the 'female'
things that they always did. Research shows that it is still women
who do the bulk of the food shopping; the food preparation and
cooking; the washing up; and the cleaning and sorting of the
fridge and larder. And, as meal times get more fragmented, with
members of the same family often eating different things at different times of the day, it is no exaggeration to say that many
women literally spend half their lives in the kitchen or dealing
with food. Little wonder, then, that they tend to eat a lot.
Remember, if it's there, we are programmed to eat it, whether it's
nibbling at food while we are preparing it or eating up the leftovers. Men aren't having it much easier, either. Whereas the
'provider' used to go out to work every day, often come home for
lunch, then return again for tea, nowadays he's probably on a
train, a plane to somewhere or driving thousands of miles a week
on the motorways. He eats on the hoof, he has business lunches,
he probably drinks too much; and he's working so hard trying to
keep ahead of the redundancy list that he hasn't time to exercise
or pay attention to his diet.

The hormone hit list   The female sex has another thing to
contend with and that is the hormone hit list. Some unlucky
women find that if they're not going through puberty, they may
have monthly PMS. If they're not having PMS they're pregnant
and the hormones have gone completely haywire; if they're not

pregnant or having PMS, they're into the menopause. The menopause brings problems from a lack of hormones sometimes, and these can contribute to overweight.

Female hormones *do* affect your behaviour and your eating patterns; they may even affect your metabolic rate. The scant or ill-informed advice most women receive on this subject is nothing short of a scandal.

I *did* tell you it's not your fault you're fat! Don't worry, in Step Three we will discover that *none* of the situations we've just looked at need make it impossible for you to get and stay slim. On closer inspection, you'll discover that either they are situations that you can alter – or, if not, you can alter your reaction to them. Fascinating? Yes.

SECTION 3:

Very Interested People

'Some people just don't seem to want me to lose weight'

Tick which statements apply to you

☐ People tell me I'm fine just as I am and I shouldn't bother with slimming.

☐ I'm often told I wasn't meant to be slim.

☐ It seems churlish to bother about my weight when there are so many more important problems in the world.

☐ Some of my women friends say it's no longer acceptable to worry about my size and I should be content with my body the way it is.

☐ I would like to lose weight but I never seem to get any real encouragement from the people closest to me.

☐ Every time I try to diet it seems to upset the people I spend most time with.

☐ My family always complain when I try to prepare lower-calorie food.

☐ I keep reading in the papers and magazines that dieting is bad for you, which is a good excuse not to diet, but I'm worried it may be true.

☐ Many members of my family are overweight and they don't seem bothered, so it's hard for me to do it alone.

It's *your* body and *your* life, yet other people seem to have a greater influence on it than you do! If you ticked many, or even one or two, of the above statements, you are letting all kinds of people stop you from losing the weight you really want to lose. I call these people VIPs – and, indeed, they may be very important in your life, but they are also very *interested*, for one reason or another, in keeping you just the way you are.

Some of the VIPs are very clever at disguising this fact. They may protest they have your best interests at heart, but this is rarely the case. The only valid reason for keeping you from getting slim and fit is that you are already slim enough and fit enough. No other reason is in your interest.

So we have to examine the motives of some of the people close to you – or, even, strangers – who are out to protect their own patches by stopping you from slimming.

People who feel guilty about their own size   If you come from an overweight family this can be an acute problem. If everyone else around is overweight it is much easier to convince yourself that that is fine. But if suddenly you become the slimmer in the camp it points up all too clearly to them the fact that: (a) being overweight isn't such a good idea and (b) it *is* possible to do something about it. So be wary of overweight family members, friends or colleagues who urge you not to slim when you know you need to: they either feel guilty enough already, or they know they will when they see the fat coming off you.

People who will feel intimidated   Losing weight means a change to the perceived order of things. Some of the people closest to you may worry that because you will *look* different you will *be* different. Partners, husbands or wives are most prone to this attitude, especially if the overweight half of the couple has a big weight problem that's been around a long time. Your partner may worry that (s)he won't be good enough for you once you are slim; or that you will be so attractive that dozens of other people will be trying to lure you away; or that you will be so much more confident that you will look for someone else as proof of your new attractiveness. If your partner has these feelings, he or she is suffering low self-esteem just as you are. People often hate change that isn't initiated by themselves, or at least they do until they realise the change isn't going to be for the worse.

Also, people don't like the idea that if you slim down, your fundamental character will change. This is why your partner and friends may be intimidated. You've always been, say, the 'fat and jolly' one, or the 'agony aunt'. If you slim, what will you be then?

And it is worth mentioning here that you yourself may have doubts too. Do you like being the jolly one? Do you love it when people tell you their troubles? *Will* slimming down make a difference to a role that you enjoy within your family or social circle?

People who will feel jealous   There are three categories of people who may be jealous if you lose weight.

1. *Unsuccessful slimmers* – for obvious reasons. You did what they couldn't do.

2. *Unsuccessful slimmers* who don't know you personally but who are getting at you through the media. First there is the 'right on' bunch of feminists who, although a tiny minority, shout with a very loud voice to tell you (if you're female) that although they reserve the right to be fat, unfit, unwashed, unshaven or whatever, it isn't fine for you to reserve *your* right to do what you choose with your body. They make you feel positively old-fashioned, out of touch, and a victim of sizeism and a male-dominated society, for even *considering* losing weight.

Second there are the scaremongers – the ones who have failed to lose weight themselves and are thus scratching around for any excuse not to try again and, of course, to justify their failure. To the scaremongers 'diet' is one of those bad four-letter words. Dieting, they maintain, is dangerous … it doesn't work … and, anyway, it's healthier to be fat.

3. *Girlfriends* (if you're female). I say girlfriends because it seems that men slimmers never have the same problem with their male friends. You may have an overweight girlfriend who doesn't want you to slim because you will no longer be on equal terms. You may have a slim girlfriend who doesn't want you to slim because suddenly you *will* be on equal terms. Slim, insecure girls often choose fat friends.

People who will worry that you're going to spoil their fun
Slimmers are often seen as spoilsports and wet blankets. Your immediate family may worry that they will feel self-conscious or sorry for you if they gorge while you nibble your lettuce. They will be worried you are going to bore them (again) with diet talk and calorie-counting. They will be alarmed that you will make them eat what you eat. Furthermore, they will hate the idea of going out anywhere with you when all you will do is drink mineral water and sit looking martyred, surrounded by other people's food, and refuse to eat a thing. You're going to spoil the fun in a big way. No wonder they can't stand the thought of you dieting. They've been there before.

People who don't want to upset you   Lastly, I expect there are a few possibly kind, possibly timid, people who know you and who realise perfectly well that you should lose some weight but who will never, ever, tell you so. They will always, if asked, look astonished and say: 'What, *you*? *You* don't need to lose weight!' These people are either terrified, for whatever reason, of upsetting you or else really think they are being kind and considerate and diplomatic in not worrying you.

We discussed in Step One how, when you are overweight, your self-esteem is likely to be low. Therefore you can be forgiven for wondering how on earth you can deal positively with all the people who seem intent on helping you to stay fat. In Step Three we will find out how to take control and lose weight *without* losing face, friends or family!

SECTION 4:

The Tyrannical Diet

'Don't mention that word "diet" to me!'

Tick which statements apply to you

☐ I'm not confident I can achieve success because I've failed so often before.

☐ I always start off on a diet with enthusiasm but soon 'tail off'.

☐ I'm either 'very good' and exist on a little or 'very bad' and binge.

☐ Dieting is so boring I don't know how anyone sticks to a diet.

☐ Diets make me miserable and depressed.

☐ The thought of having to go on another diet makes me feel as though I've got to take an exam.

☐ If I cheat even once on a diet and eat something not allowed, that's it, I give up.

☐ I can't get down to the amount I used to weigh in my teens no matter how hard I try.

☐ I never lose weight as quickly as I want to.

☐ I've spent a fortune on diet products and still I'm fat.

If you ticked some, or many, of these statements, you are undoubtedly a victim of the diet mentality – largely a state brought about by sections of the diet industry which make you believe that dieting is a form of self-imposed torture to be endured if you have the strength, a battle to be won or lost; by a diet industry which persuades you to adopt the 'all or nothing' approach – feast or fast, win or lose, good or bad, fat or thin, right or wrong.

There is a vast array of people – many of them women – in the UK who have spent years and years trapped in the misery of the diet mentality. Stuck in a trap not really of their own making, they start diets that end too soon, or they lose weight then put every ounce back on again.

You're probably one of them. I expect you've tried slimming pills – if not on prescription, then through mail order or from the health-food shop or the chemist. Pills that promised to help you burn up calories as you slept, or to dull your appetite; slimming potions, slimming biscuits, slimming drinks to save the bother of having to make yourself a proper meal; miracle diets cut out of magazines or papers suggesting you eat only bananas and eggs, or cheese and grapefruit, or nothing but carbohydrates at one meal and then protein at the next. Have you tried slimming clinics, slimming patches, slimming ear clips, slimming sauna suits, slimming wax treatments, slimming creams or the 'negative calories' diet?

If you have and you're still just as fat as, or probably fatter than, you were to start with, well, you can be forgiven for believing the people who tell you 'diets don't work'.

Even if you've tried none of the above methods, you've probably still been on and off more diet programmes than you care to remember – and you're still overweight. No matter how good your intentions, the diet always gets you in the end; it's too boring, too mean, too miserable, too deprivational, too hard. And every time you give up the fight, the next attempt is even harder. It isn't because 'dieting makes you fat'. It's because dieting makes you fed up.

As with fashion, the diet industry tends to encourage false expectations of what can be achieved. I have seen advertisements that, with 'before' and 'after' pictures, appear to show a

16-stone (101.6 kg) person shrinking to 9 stone (57.2 kg) in a matter of weeks. I am constantly appalled at the pathetic, painfully thin models used by fashion editors and designers to 'show off' designer clothes, with the result that many women feel that they, too, ought to be that thin. I have also been horrified time and again at the images of perfection adorning many diet products. The quest to lose that last ounce, to become 'perfect', is a sad road leading only to frustration and failure for most of us.

The diet mentality has helped you to fail, not to win, because *it made you try too hard*. Diets that require you to be too 'good' will, ultimately and inevitably, make you 'bad'. The 'success or failure' approach means there is no middle ground, no room for manoeuvre. And it is this mentality that can permanently keep you in a state of either 'dieting' or 'not dieting', a state of never being relaxed and happy about eating – just resentful when you're dieting and guilty when you're not. Dieting like this is a bleak, unproductive and totally unnecessary process.

To get slim for life, you need to get out of this diet trap. In Step Three we will be exploring ways to do just that. We will be reducing the importance of 'Diet' (with a capital D) in your life. We will be reshaping your attitude to weight loss and what *you* can achieve, and looking at the 'good guys' of the slimming industry – the ones who *can* help.

STEP TWO ROUND-UP

Are you ready to move on?
So now, at last, you know *why* you overeat – and for most of us there is not just one reason – but many. Often the very last of those reasons is hunger or nutritional needs.

What we will be doing in Step Three is encouraging you to become strong enough to eat, at least on most occasions, for the *right* reasons – a feat that would have been impossible if you had not worked your way through Step Two.

Now, before we move on, I want you to go back and find that list of motivating factors that you drew up at the end of Step One. Sit down and go through them slowly. Think hard about each objective. Picture yourself slimmer, focus really strongly on you as a slim person doing what it is you want to do, e.g., zipping up a pair of jeans or diving into the swimming pool. Savour the images you create. Now answer the following questions:

☐ Are you fully aware of *why* you have put on weight, *why* you have stayed overweight and *why* you have failed to lose weight?

☐ Are you looking forward to Step Three where together we can formulate your own sensible strategies for overcoming those shape saboteurs?

☐ Can you picture yourself slim for life?

Yes? Then here we go – but remember, be patient. *You are already on your slimming campaign*. The slimming started when you began Step One.

STEP THREE
Take Control

Begin to be slim for life!

Step Three is probably *the* most vital part of your Slim For Life campaign, because it is here that you will learn that you do have the ability to control your eating habits and, therefore, can take lasting control of your weight.

What do I mean by 'control', though? Don't think of being in control as being rigid, inflexible or obsessive. Those are all negative forms of control which usually indicate that you are a victim of the 'tyrannical diet', still trying too hard and expecting too much of yourself.

No, when you take control of your eating you are simply making decisions and choices and sometimes making changes, because *you* want to. You can and should be relaxed, happy and realistic about what you can achieve, not uptight.

Control means, for instance, making the decision to be more focused on what you want to achieve. It means deciding to be more assertive and less passive, more conscious of what you can do to help your body and less fatalistic.

Control means, where it's feasible, taking charge of your life. The saboteur situations we discussed in Step Two aren't all going to disappear overnight, so what we're going to do in Step Three is deal with them. It may take time, especially if your self-confidence is low, but as we work through the sections your self-esteem will improve along with your ability to control your diet, so all the time the task grows easier. Never doubt that:

YOU CAN TAKE DECISIONS

YOU CAN MAKE CHOICES

YOU CAN MAKE CHANGES

YOU CAN BE SLIM

USING STEP THREE

There are four sections that follow, each one relating, in order, to the four sections – and sets of statements – in Step Two. If you ticked any of the statements in any of those four sections in Step Two, you should read the corresponding section here and cover all the exercises in it.

Even if one or more sections in Step Two contain statements you didn't tick, I nevertheless recommend that you read through the corresponding section(s) here because I am sure you will find it interesting and enlightening.

Work through the sections in order from 1 to 4, working on only one at a time. Spend a week or more on section 1. So, if you have to work through all four sections, it will take you probably two to three weeks. You can spend longer if you need to. Don't feel impatient. Remember, this may not be a conventional diet but conventional diets haven't worked for you; this method *will*, if you trust it. It is vital not to skip Step Three and it is vital not to skip through it. I shall tell you something very encouraging: you may well find that, while you are working your way through the Step Three sections, you are losing weight anyway. Because what we are doing together *is* working on your fat! Also, let me remind you again about all the time you've wasted on previous diets or in worrying about your weight. Time spent on Step Three is productive time that will not only help you to get slim easily but will give you the foundation for lifelong slimness.

When you have finished all the sections in Step Three, turn to page 150 and read the round-up.

For the Step Three sections you will need:

- A pen
- A notebook
- Some quiet time to yourself

SECTION 1:

Take a New Look at Food

In Step Two, section one showed you that many of your poorer eating habits are a direct result both of the way society has changed in recent years and of the persuasive food industry.

You have overeaten too many of the foods – fats and sugars (and perhaps alcohol) – that tend to make us fat and along the way you have become convinced that these were the foods you really enjoy.

Now I am going to show you easy ways to, literally, tip the scales in your body's favour; how to keep the pleasure in eating without involving all the unnecessary calories; how to get along with food in a slightly different way.

'I don't really eat much, yet I'm fat.'
'However much I cut down on food,
I can't lose weight.'

Overweight people tell me time after time that they can't lose weight on a diet. They will tell me, say, that even though they are only eating 1,000 calories a day they aren't shedding an ounce.

Yet in every trial conducted where people were put in controlled conditions and fed 1,000 calories a day, they *all* lost weight. Lots of it. A recent report has backed up what I already knew: that very many would-be dieters eat and drink masses more than they think they are eating and drinking. The truth is that unless you know what you're doing it is possible to *appear* to be eating little when in fact you are eating quite a lot.

Old-style versus new-style eating

Here's an example of a typical day's 'hardly eating anything' that *won't result in the average woman losing any weight at all.*

Breakfast
Large glass fruit juice
Small helping (60 g, 2¼ oz) muesli with milk to cover

Lunch
Small piece (approx. 50 g, 2 oz) Cheddar
with 2 cream crackers very lightly buttered
1 tomato, little lettuce
1 fruit yogurt

Dinner
1 small lamb chop
1 small baked potato with small knob butter
Small portion mixed peas and carrots
Small portion (approx. 75 g, 3 oz) ice cream
topped with 2 teaspoons chopped mixed nuts

Throughout day
Coffee or tea with milk, no sugar

This is a day's consumption that, to the 'dieter', will seem very little on the plate, but in fact it is not only very high in fat and low in carbohydrates (the complete opposite of a good, long-term healthy diet) but also contains in the region of 1,900 calories – about the amount of calories an average woman taking little exercise will consume in an average day. If calorie intake equals calorie output, there will be no weight gain – but no loss, either!

And yet, eating like that, the consumer is under the impression she *is* dieting and feels cross that there are no results. *No* bread! *No* pastry! *No* chocolate! *No* alcohol! *No* sugar in her coffee! *No* fried foods! *No* between-meal snacks! She's been so good, she feels, by sticking to fruit juice, healthy muesli, crisp-breads and small portions of everything.

One of the first keys to successful weight loss and weight maintenance is *knowledge*. The 'dieter' illustrated above lacks knowledge about the fat-rich foods.

These were her main mistakes that day:

- Using full-cream milk on cereal and in drinks.
- Muesli is denser than most cereals and contains more fat. Even a small bowlful will be much higher in calories than a larger helping of most other cereals.
- Cheddar cheese is a very high-fat food. Cream crackers are quite high in fat, too – and butter, even lightly spread, adds many more calories.
- Fruit yogurt can be low in fat and calories, but not always. Some contain whole milk, added sugar and even added cream.
- Lamb chops, unless very well trimmed, are a high-fat meat. Even grilling doesn't help a lot, unless you remove the visible fat.
- That small knob of butter on the potato could contain almost as many calories as the potato itself. Fats are easy to miscalculate as they are dense, high-calorie foods.
- Ice cream is a reasonable dessert but even a few nuts add on lots of fat and calories. Almost all nuts are very high in fat.

This is what I call the 'old-fashioned British' style of eating that has contributed towards our weight problem. With a bit more knowledge, this woman could halve the fat and calories in her day's eating *without* substantially changing the type of food she eats, *without* feeling hungry, and yet *with* more food actually on the plate and *with* between-meal snacks too. She will also be giving herself a much, much healthier diet as she slims down.

Here's that same day's eating converted at least partially to the 'new style' – the style we should aim for to get slim.

Breakfast
1 piece fresh fruit
Medium helping flaked cereal (any kind except with
added sugar) with skimmed milk to cover

Mid-morning
1 banana

Lunch
40 g (1½ oz) half-fat Cheddar-style cheese
with 1 slice wholemeal bread with a little low-fat spread
Large salad
1 low-fat diet fruit yogurt

Dinner
1 small extra-lean lamb fillet steak, grilled
1 large baked potato topped with 2 teaspoons fromage frais
Large portion fresh peas
Large portion carrots
Medium portion reduced-fat ice cream
or ice cream substitute

Throughout day
Coffee or tea with skimmed milk

I have come to the conclusion after years of seeing other types
of diet at work – and, largely, failing – that any form of dieting
other than getting into the habit of eating a healthy, lower-fat,
higher-carbohydrate diet is for most people a total waste of
time.

You don't need to have less *food on your plate, you need to
make* swops – *swops that, mostly, you won't even notice.*

In Step Four you will be learning more about fats and carbohydrates and how to balance them in a slimming diet. But for
now it is important that you take stock of your current diet,
identify where you are going wrong and begin to make some
decisions about how best to alter the balance in a way that suits
you.

Why do fats make us fat?

There are five main reasons why fat is the chief culprit in making and keeping us fat.

1. *At 9 calories per gram, it has more than double the calories of a gram of protein (4 calories per gram) or carbohydrate (3.75 calories per gram).* Fat, protein and carbohydrate are the only kinds of constituents in our diet (apart from alcohol, which contains 7 calories per gram) that give us calories. All the other things we eat and drink (water, vitamins, minerals, fibre, micronutrients) contain no calories. Put simply, weight for weight, fat is higher in calories than any other food.

2. *The body likes to convert fat in our food into fat on ourselves.* All the latest research shows that spare fat in your diet – i.e., that not used for your energy needs – is much more easily laid down as body fat than carbohydrate is. Backing up this research, an American experiment found that people who ate a high-carbohydrate but low-fat diet lost weight steadily without decreasing their overall food intake.

3. *When you eat fat, the natural, weight-regulating body mechanisms don't appear to work properly.* Research carried out by much respected Andrew Prentice of the Medical Research Council at the Dunn Nutrition Unit in Cambridge has recently made two interesting discoveries about how our bodies react to fat when we eat it. First, he believes that, because most people's body-fat stores are so large (over 100,000 calories' worth of fat on an average woman's body), when we eat fat the body doesn't 'notice' and therefore doesn't send out the normal signals of appetite being sated. Whereas if you eat carbohydrate, then because the body's carbo stores are *low* – about 1,000 calories' worth – the body quickly notices that it is being bombarded with, say, double the quantities it can store and sends up an 'I am full' message to the brain.

His second discovery revealed that when we eat protein, carbohydrate or alcohol, our body metabolism speeds up and begins to burn off extra calories. But when we eat fat, it doesn't. Its rate stays the same.

4. *Fat makes other foods more palatable.* When fats are mixed with other foods, as in many commercially made products or in home baking, for instance, you eat much more than you would have done if the food had consisted simply of the other ingredients. Sugar not mixed with fat is hard to eat in quantity. Think of a meringue (just sugar and egg white): how much could you eat at one sitting? But combine sugar with fat – in, say, a slice of cream cake – and you can eat much more. Fats, probably because they melt in your mouth, make it very easy to slip down hundreds of extra calories. Apply that to a baked potato. It seems to be much easier to eat with a huge knob of butter than it is on its own. Dry bread you will eat until you feel full, but spread it with butter and you will probably eat two or three times as much. Fats in and on food make us eat *more*.

5. *Fat is easy to miscalculate.* On most slimming diets, dieters are requested to weigh and measure quantities but, research shows, people tend to guess, at least after the first day or two on a diet. With less dense items, such as bread or vegetables, that doesn't matter much because a miscalculation between, say, 25 g (1 oz) and 40 g (1½ oz) of bread means only an extra thirty or so calories. But if you miscalculate between, say, 25 g (1 oz) and 40 g (1½ oz) of butter, you are eating an extra 105 calories! This fat miscalculation is probably another reason why dieters who think they are on a low-calorie diet don't lose any weight.

So now you can see why it is so important to get down the fat levels in your diet if you are to lose weight successfully and keep it off. And, so that you don't go hungry existing on small meals, you need to replace the fat with carbohydrate. A simple way to understand the difference between the old-fashioned 'fattening' way of eating and the new-style 'slim' way of eating is to think of what you eat in terms of a pyramid.

You can see from these pyramids how the two diets compare:

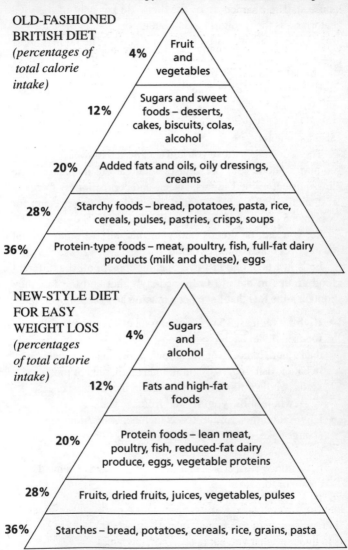

OLD-FASHIONED BRITISH DIET
(percentages of total calorie intake)

4% Fruit and vegetables

12% Sugars and sweet foods – desserts, cakes, biscuits, colas, alcohol

20% Added fats and oils, oily dressings, creams

28% Starchy foods – bread, potatoes, pasta, rice, cereals, pulses, pastries, crisps, soups

36% Protein-type foods – meat, poultry, fish, full-fat dairy products (milk and cheese), eggs

NEW-STYLE DIET FOR EASY WEIGHT LOSS
(percentages of total calorie intake)

4% Sugars and alcohol

12% Fats and high-fat foods

20% Protein foods – lean meat, poultry, fish, reduced-fat dairy produce, eggs, vegetable proteins

28% Fruits, dried fruits, juices, vegetables, pulses

36% Starches – bread, potatoes, cereals, rice, grains, pasta

At first glance, the old-fashioned British diet may not look too bad. The broad base of the diet – 36 per cent of the total calories – is the 'protein foods', but unfortunately they are also mostly high-fat, or relatively high-fat, foods. The fat in most of these foods accounts for between a third and three-quarters of their total calories! As for the 'starch group', well, bread, potatoes, pasta and rice are fine, yes, but our current carbohydrate intake consists of a very high proportion of the refined starches found in bakery goods, such as sweet and savoury pastries that also include fat.

The added fats – those you add at table and in cooking – alone comprise another 20 per cent of total calorie intake; and the low-nutrient refined sugars, sweets and confectionery form the rest, along with fresh fruits and vegetables, which account for less than 5 per cent of many people's calorie intake each day!

So, you see, fat creeps into your diet, almost unnoticed, in nearly every area of the pyramid.

Let's just take one last eye-opening look at all the different food groups in the old-fashioned-style diet and the fats they contain – the fats that have been making and keeping you fat.

- High-fat (at least 35 per cent of total calories) 'protein' foods include: bacon, beef (most kinds), chicken with skin, duck, ham, lamb, liver, meat loaf, pork, sausages, pâté, fish in batter, fish fingers, scampi, tuna in oil, nuts of most kinds, whole milk, all cheeses except diet cottage cheese, eggs, whole-milk yogurts and fromage frais.
- High-fat 'carbohydrate' foods include: chips, doughnuts, sponge cake, croissants, scones, biscuits of most kinds, cereal bars, oatcakes, pasties, most kinds of pastry, jam tarts, mince pies, crisps and savoury snacks and canned cream of tomato soup.
- High-fat 'added fat' foods include: butter, margarine, low-fat spreads, polyunsaturated spreads, all cooking oils, all salad oils, all mayonnaises, all types of cream, French dressing, salad cream, tartare sauce and white sauce.

- High-fat sweet, dessert and confectionery foods include: chocolate of all kinds, standard ice cream (dairy or non-dairy), custard and rice puddings, gâteaux, cheesecakes, fruit pies.
- Many savoury recipe dishes, home-made or bought ready-made, including soups, casseroles, lasagnes, sauces, moussakas, curries, chilli, satay, stews and casseroles.

In the rest of this section, and in Step Four, I shall be helping you to adapt your diet in order to minimise the fat content of all these foods – so that you can still enjoy them, but in the context of a 'new style' diet rather than in the old-fashioned British way. With some careful adaptations and 'swops', we will be able to get the proportions in your diet to reflect the 'new-style' pyramid on page 67 – a pyramid that remains valid whether you want to lose weight or simply to maintain your weight loss.

The new-style pyramid places a much greater emphasis on the natural (or nearly natural) high-carbohydrate foods: bread, potatoes, grains of all kinds – including rice – breakfast cereals and pasta. It places almost as much emphasis on fruits, dried fruits, vegetables and pulses. All these foods in the two groups are the 'complex carbohydrates' that together will form the bulk of your diet. (Pulses, by the way, are also high-protein foods, but for the purposes of our new-style pyramid they are best included with the two vegetable and starch groups.)

Our protein needs aren't great – about 10 to 15 per cent of calories in our total diet – so in keeping the meat, fish and dairy-produce part of the pyramid to 20 per cent of total calories and by retaining in this group only the reasonably low-fat items (such as white fish, poultry with no skin and the reduced-fat versions of milk and cheese), we ensure that in adding protein to the diet you are not by default adding too much extra fat. In this protein group I include the new vegetable-protein foods, such as TVP (soya protein), Quorn and tofu, all of which are reasonably low-fat sources of protein.

I estimate that at least 10 per cent of the calories in this food group will be fat calories; the other 10 per cent will be protein. (Protein is also present in the complex-carbohydrate group of foods; bread, rice and so on all have reasonable amounts and even fruit and vegetables have a little. So, in all, the new-style diet will easily meet protein needs.)

Near the top of the new-style pyramid are the fats you add in recipes and at table; the very high-fat foods such as dressings and cream; and all the other high-fat foods featured lower down in the old-style diet but not in this pyramid, e.g., pastries and baked foods.

The tip of the new pyramid allows for sugars and alcohol. These last two groups at the top of the pyramid joined together amount to 16 per cent of the total calorie intake and compose the fatty, sugary foods we should be cutting down on.

*   *   *

'But I like fat and all those fatty foods.'

So now you know (perhaps you already did know, but it is surprising, even after ten years of being told to 'eat less fat', how many people *don't* know just where that fat is lurking) that the main reason you are overweight is because you've been eating more fat than you realised, and that to cut down you need to change somewhat the way you eat. But you can't see how you're going to live with that. Well, this is where we find out.

Think back to Step Two. There you learnt that your eating habits and 'preferences' have been largely foisted upon you over the years by social conditioning. It is relatively easy, once you have decided that you want to take control, to undo that conditioning.

An American university research study, and other experiments, concluded that the taste for fatty foods can be disposed of very quickly. A thousand women reduced their fat intake to

25 per cent or less (after a previous norm of about 40 per cent or more, in line with many Americans and British). After six months on this low-fat diet, the women reported that they now actually disliked high-fat foods. Side effects from switching to a high-fat diet from a low-fat diet include severe indigestion, heartburn, constipation and chronic lethargy – as well as immediate weight gain.

Here then, are my own tried and tested ways to help you reduce the fat in your diet, along with some suggested experiments for you to carry out yourself.

THE EASIEST WAYS TO CUT FAT

- Make changes gradually.
- Make swops in what you buy.
- Make swops in how you cook.
- Alter the balance on your plate.
- Make changes you are most able to live with.
- Incorporate into your diet sensible amounts of what you can't live without.

Make changes gradually

Although the 'kill or cure' approach works for some people, usually the best method for change is 'little by little'. Also, as your digestive system takes time to adapt to a different diet, this makes sense physically as well as emotionally. And it makes sense in a third way: your palate will then painlessly adapt to what you offer it.

Here are a couple of examples of making changes gradually rather than quickly:

You decide to cut down on fat by using skimmed milk instead of whole milk. But your palate tells you you dislike the skimmed milk in your tea and on your cereals: it doesn't 'taste right'. So you go back to your whole milk. *What you should have done* was choose semi-skimmed milk as a compromise for a few weeks and then tried the fully skimmed.

You decide that one of the reasons your fat intake is high is your love of biscuits, so you determine to cut them out. But after a day or two you are craving biscuits, so you start eating them even more avidly than before. *What you should have done* was either replace your biscuits with a lower-fat, lower-calorie kind (if possible) or cut down the number (perhaps by buying them individually wrapped).

Make changes gradually so you have time to get accustomed to them in every way. After a time they are incorporated into your life as if they are habits you have always had.

Make swops in what you buy

Although it is the case, as I explained in Step Two, that you are, largely (perhaps *very* largely!), what the food industry has made you, the good news is that if we show the food industry – through what we buy in the supermarkets – that what we want is lower fat, lower sugar, healthier produce, then eventually that message will get through and the shelves will reflect our wishes.

That means making a determined and wholesale effort to shop the new-style pyramid way. Since there is only profit to be made in manufacturing and selling packets of cream cakes or trifle mixes and the like if the products disappear from the shop shelves, any line that sits there for too long gets replaced by something that *will* sell.

Already all the supermarkets and most of the smaller shops are offering reduced-fat, reduced-sugar, reduced-calorie versions of high-fat, high-cal, high-sugar foods, yet still it is frequently more difficult for us to locate these lines than the traditional versions. However, the most popular of the reduced-fat items, the ones with which we are very familiar, are big sellers and are therefore stocked just as prominently as their counterparts, skimmed milk and reduced-fat spreads being the two that come to mind first.

The following are all swops that will save masses of fat calories. Tick all the swops that are new to you and try out one or two of them every time you do a shop.

☐ **Low-fat spread instead of butter/ordinary margarine**
Yes, low-fat spread is a high-fat food, but it contains only half the fat (or less) of the conventional spreads and it tends to spread thinner, too. If you have tried low-fat spread before and not liked it, pick a small size of a different brand, because taste quality varies enormously and some are very pleasant indeed.

☐ **Low-fat yogurt instead of whole-milk yogurt** Read the labels to make sure that the yogurt you buy really is low in fat; some aren't.

☐ **Lower-fat cheeses instead of traditional cheeses** More and more reduced-fat varieties, such as Cheddar, Edam, Cheshire, Red Leicester, processed slices, soft cream-type cheeses, cheese spreads, roulé and cottage, are available and many of the traditional cheeses are lower in fat and calories than other varieties. For instance, Brie and Camembert have less fat and fewer calories (about 85 per 25 g, 1 oz) than cream cheese or Cambozola (110 per 25 g, 1 oz). Practise reading the labels and comparing the fat contents of the various cheeses.

Cheddar addicts often don't like the reduced-fat imitation varieties (again, some are better than others). If that includes you, here are three tips: (1) the reduced-fat versions are fine in cooking, (2) if you buy a very strong Cheddar (e.g., mature farmhouse or extra mature) you will probably find that half your normal amount suffices because the strong varieties are much more flavoursome than the mild Cheddars, and (3) grated cheese goes further.

☐ **Lean cuts of meat instead of the traditional cuts** Due to demand, leaner meat is being produced all the time, but even so I still see a lot of very fatty cuts of meat in the butchers' and supermarkets. Ignore those and always go for the extra-lean cuts that are labelled as such. Many people don't choose these because they are more expensive, but if you buy the cheaper cuts and then have to cut the fat off (or throw melted fat away after cooking) it is false economy. Not only that, but by buying the lean cuts you remove the temptation to eat the fat rather than throw it away.

You can get lean mince, lean trimmed chops, lean bacon, low-fat sausages and low-fat ham.

☐ **Tuna in brine instead of tuna in oil**　Tuna in oil is a high-fat food; tuna in brine is a very low-fat food. If you like tuna it's an easy swop to make.

☐ **Straight-cut, thick-cut chips instead of crinkled chips or thin-cut chips**　Crinkled and/or thin chips absorb much more fat than straight and thick-cut chips, so if you are a chip addict the fat- and calorie-saving can be great. Oven chips are a good bet, too; as brands vary, go for the ones that contain least fat.

☐ **Low-fat crisps instead of regular crisps**　The saving per pack isn't much, but if you're very partial to crisps it could make a difference.

☐ **Spraying oil instead of cooking oil**　You can now buy a special spray-on oil that gives the pan a very light coating for 'frying' without adding calories.

☐ **Extra-thick single cream or fromage frais or Greek-style yogurt instead of double cream.**

☐ **'Alternative to cream'** (half the fat) **or cream in an aerosol container** (because it contains so much air that a big 'squirt' works out at minimal calories) **instead of single cream.**

☐ **Lower-fat dressings instead of full-fat versions** These almost all taste fine, so swop full-fat mayonnaise for a reduced-calorie type. Salad cream, Thousand Island, tartare and French dressing are available in no- or low-cal versions.

☐ **Lower-fat proteins instead of high-fat proteins** Make the decision to base more main-course dishes on the lower-fat protein foods such as lean chicken, turkey, veal (if you will eat it), Quorn, white fish and pulses. Cod contains 8 per cent fat calories, while steak (without the fat border on it) has 32 per cent fat calories. So if you're a red-meat fan, say, decide to give up one red-meat meal a week to start with. Further on in this chapter, and in Step Four, you will find many ideas for making lower-fat meals just as interesting, tasty and satisfying as high-fat meals.

Make swops in how you cook

You can cut out even more fat from your cooking by using the following methods. Again, tick all those that are new to you and aim regularly to try out each one.

☐ **Dry-fry, don't deep-fry** Many things that you used to fry can nowadays be oven-baked, but, if you don't want to do that, the next best thing is to dry-fry. You need a good, heavy-bottomed, non-stick frying pan and a tiny brushing of oil (or the new spray-on oil). Once the pan is heated, many foods, from fish to sauté potatoes, can be cooked this way.

☐ **Grill fatty foods, don't fry them** You'll cut out even more fat calories if you grill, say, a slice of bacon over a slatted splash guard so that the fat in the meat melts, runs through the slats and is easy to discard. Grill foods such as bacon and sausages until really well done in order to eliminate even more fat.

☐ **Experiment with methods that reduce the fat or oil content in your favourite recipes** Many new-style recipes for you to try are included in Step Four, but almost any recipe can be adapted in a similar way. For instance, if you're browning onions or meat for a casserole, you could reduce the specified fat or oil down to nearly nothing, especially if you use non-stick cookware. Also, many soup recipes suggest frying the vegetables first in oil, but you can usually omit this step and simply simmer them in stock before blending.

☐ **If you're using mince in a recipe, pour off any fat that rises to the top** (or use a fat-absorbing brush to lift it off).

☐ **Casseroles can be made in advance,** left in the fridge and then any solid fat that appears on the top is easily removed.

☐ Use **reduced-fat cooking spread** for baking.

All these things are easy to do and won't detract from the taste of your cooking at all.

Alter the balance on your plate

Get into the habit of 'thinking pyramid' every time you make up a plateful of food for yourself. See how often you can compose a meal of which the largest part is complex carbohydrates from the base of the pyramid and the next largest is from the fruit and veg section, followed by a smaller-than-usual portion of your protein food and a little bit of something fatty.

Old-style balance Large steak or slices of roast meat; medium portion of potatoes; big knob of butter on both potatoes and steak; small portion of peas.

New-style balance Much smaller steak or slices of roast meat; much larger portion of potatoes; at least two helpings of vegetables; a very small knob of butter on the potatoes, and fat-free gravy over the rest of the plate to avoid dryness.

Keep looking back at that pyramid and get the balance right! *It will take time,* but don't worry about this.

You can alter the balance in other ways, too. Instead of that steak-and-potatoes meal, try one that is based on carbohydrates – say, a big plate of spaghetti or rice topped with a vegetable stir-fry containing just a very *little* meat.

Make changes you are most able to live with

Some of the suggestions I make may seem more easy, more pleasant and more practical to you than others. Work first on the ones that seem easiest. Everyone is different; your diet doesn't have to be exactly the same as everyone else's. Your preferences matter. If you don't take account of them you won't succeed in losing weight and keeping it off. You're not being asked to sacrifice everything you hold dear, but only to look and see if there are ways of improving your diet and to understand that your taste in food can alter.

If, after giving something – say, low-fat spread – a fair trial, you just can't get on with it, well, don't worry, you don't *have* to eat low-fat spread to get slim.

Incorporate into your diet sensible amounts of what you can't live without

If there is something you crave, at least for now have it in sensible amounts. If you are cutting down on fats in general, incorporating my ideas into your daily diet – and incorporating more as you go along – then you can eat your one, two or three very favourite high-fat foods without feeling guilty. I will show you in Step Four how to judge what 'sensible amounts' mean in your case.

By the time you have worked your way through all of Step Three you should find, in any event, that you are much more able to control the *amount* you eat of the high-fat foods.

ACTION

1. Now make a list in your notepad of the fat-reducing things you are going to try and/or to buy. Put them in an order that appeals to you – then go ahead and turn the words into action.

2. Walk round your largest local supermarket and see how many reduced-fat products you can find that you hadn't noticed before.

3. Practise reading the nutrition labels and compare the fat contents of similar products per 100 g. Be aware, though, that the stated percentages for the fat contents of foods will be misleadingly low because the weight of the water contained (surprisingly high, even for solid foods such as cheese and meat) means that the fat-content percentage is correspondingly reduced. Cheddar cheese, for instance, contains over 74 per cent fat calories and 25 per cent protein calories (no carbohydrate calories) but the label won't state '74% fat'; instead it will probably say something like 'per 100 g: 33% fat; 26% protein'. The missing 40-plus per cent is water, which is calorie-free.

However, bearing this in mind, what you can do is compare different products for relative fat values. If on a cheese, say, '10% fat' is stated, you'll know it has much less fat than a cheese that states '33% fat'.

4. Just for interest, try this taste test. You reckon you really like fat? Well, get some teaspoons. Fill one with butter, one with margarine, one with lard, one with suet and one with vegetable oil (e.g. corn or sunflower oil). Now shut your eyes and, one by one, eat those spoonfuls of fat. (No need to hurry. Take your time. Savour each mouthful. Take plenty of time between sampling.)

Done it? Now write here your honest opinion of those fats. Did you enjoy them? If not, how did they make you feel?

Butter ....

Margarine ....

Lard ....

Suet ....

Vegetable oil ....

I can't tell exactly what you've put, but I wouldn't mind betting that alongside at least some of those spoonfuls are comments that have surprised you.

5. Here's another exercise. Pick whichever of the above fats you enjoyed *most* (or, should I say, disliked least) and put a big chunk (or bowl, if it's liquid) of it in front of you. Now take a spoon, sit down and eat as much of that fat as you can in one go. Go on – now!

Right. Finished? How much did you manage to eat? Again, I can't be sure, but I bet it was very little.

Fat on its own, you see, isn't all that terrific. In fact, there is nothing truly wonderful about fat; nothing so glorious that you can't live with less. *Why have you been letting such a boring thing as fat keep you fat all this time?*

Many other fatty foods that you are used to eating are also not that special if you approach them with an unblinkered eye and a clear palate. I did that with chips. I used to consider a mound of them the ultimate indulgence because, in my head, they were 'naughty, forbidden' foods. When I recognised the fact that most chips are pretty flabby, rather soggy and often any flavour attached can be attributed only to the liberal amounts of salt, vinegar or tomato ketchup that is put on them, I realised I didn't actually like chips very much at all. Nowadays I'm content to take a trip to McDonalds once in a blue moon just for a bag of their chips, which to my mind are the only ones worth eating! I enjoy every mouthful and, because these chips are only an occasional treat, I don't feel guilty.

6. *Keep a 'fat diary'.* In the week ahead, try to adopt this approach to everything you eat that has a high-fat content (refer back to the list on pages 68–69). Take, say, a meat pasty;

concentrate on how you feel when you're eating it and afterwards report that reaction in your notebook and rate the enjoyment you got from it on a scale of 1 (least enjoyment) to 10
(most enjoyment). At the end of a week in which you have kept
up this exercise, you will know that the foods that rated the low-
est scores will be the ones to 'work on' – to cut down on, or to
cut out and replace with lower-fat alternatives.

I'd also like you to think about *why* you were eating those
things in the first place and to write in your reasons next to the
enjoyment score. If the enjoyment score was high, your reason
may simply be 'because I wanted it'! But if the score was lower
or low, your reasons may range from 'I dashed into my local
shop to buy something for supper and got the pasty [or whatev-
er] because it was the only thing I could eat straight away without having to cook' or, perhaps, 'Everyone else was eating
pasties so that's what I had to eat too', to, maybe, 'I've always
eaten pasties; I just didn't think about it'.

As you are discovering, we eat for all kinds of reasons – and
perhaps you don't like fat as much as you think you do. What
you need to do, if your Fat Diary reveals remarks like those
above, is read on through the rest of section one – then sections
two and three as well, to help you control these other factors.

But, meanwhile, I want you to add one last thing to your Fat
Diary and that is: for each 'fat food' that didn't rate very highly,
your own idea for reducing that item in your diet. Say, you ate a
fatty pork chop and didn't really enjoy the fatty part of it. You
will put: 'Buy lean choice, extra-trimmed, next time' or, even:
'In future consider choosing some pork fillet to make a stir-fry
with rice.'

I would like you to carry on keeping your Fat Diary in the weeks
ahead. As you gain control over the least-favourite items, you
can then begin working on the favourite items, too. As I said
before, if there is an item you really do love then you don't have
to give it up: you can build it into your diet and still lose weight

A day of your Fat Diary should look something like this:

Date/time	Food eaten	Score	Reason	Solution
Mon. 6th 9 a.m.	Sausage roll	4 (bit chewy)	Hungry on way to work as didn't have time for breakfast	Make list of quick, easy things for breakfast
5.30 p.m.	Bar of chocolate	8	Bought paper on way home, saw the choc display and couldn't resist	Buy smallest bar possible next time

and stay slim. However, it is always worth finding out if there is any lower-fat alternative to your high-fat delight. For instance, if you really do enjoy a savoury pie, well, have you ever tried filo pastry? You do the brushing-on of fat or oil yourself and if you're careful you can halve the fat in a pastry topping without losing any taste. If you adore butter: remember to take it out of the fridge so it spreads thinner, or else buy the spreadable butter now available. If you're crazy about cheese sauce, look up the recipe section in Step Four and you'll find you can reduce the fat in that sauce greatly with no loss of flavour.

Always ask yourself: 'Can I make a swop that won't deprive me of the taste I like?' If you always do this – and I trust you to – if you keep that image of the new-style pyramid in your mind all the time and make a real effort to alter the balance of the food on your plate, you will gradually alter how you feel about food, you will alter your palate and your expectations of your diet – and you will lose weight. You'll also be doing your health a big favour by reducing fats.

*   *   *

'I've always had a sweet tooth, though. Isn't it sweet things rather than fat that are keeping me fat?'

Sweet tastes are something we are, literally, born to enjoy. Breast milk is sweet; so is formula milk. By the time we are weaned, the taste for sweet foods is well established. Both breast and formula milks also contain fat and it's this seductive combination of sugar and fat that is, I believe, the main problem.

Sugar, on its own, isn't irresistible. You can carry out a taste test similar to the one for fat described earlier. Place a sugar bowl in front of you and see how much of the sugar you can eat, by itself, before having to admit defeat. It won't be much. It's just too sweet! Nobody gets fat through a weakness for confectionery that doesn't contain fat – boiled sweets, for instance, or fruit pastilles. The sweet items that most people crave, and that give them a weight problem, are the fat-laden ones like chocolate (which we'll come to in a minute), cakes, biscuits, cheesecakes, pastries and creamy desserts.

In fact our national consumption of packet sugars – e.g. granulated – has halved in recent years. But, although increasing numbers of us are drinking tea and coffee without adding sugar and using less sugar on cereal, there has been a massive increase in our consumption of those hidden sugars in the items listed above.

We should try to reduce the amount of sugary foods that we eat for three main reasons:

1. The combination of fat and sugar in most sweet foods will make you eat even if you aren't hungry. (For more on hunger versus appetite, see page 108.) You will be inclined to eat puddings, desserts and snacks which literally 'slip down' before you have really noticed.

2. Sugar, in all its forms – white, brown, glucose, syrup, fructose – contains carbohydrate but little else. Even honey and molasses contain very few other nutrients: no vitamins, no minerals, but approximately 100 calories per 25 g (1 oz). So if you eat a lot of the high-sugar items at the expense of more nutritious foods, your diet may lack vital nutrients.

3. Simple sugars, with the exception of fructose (fruit sugar), are not so effective in curbing hunger as are the complex carbohydrates. They are more quickly absorbed into the bloodstream, so, at first, you will feel full. But, as the sugar is so rapidly dealt with, this blood-glucose level quickly sinks, leaving you feeling hungry again soon.

However, for sweet-toothers, all is not lost! Although, as with fat, experiments have shown that it is possible to conquer a desire for sweet foods as quickly as it is to overcome a taste for fatty ones, you needn't go cold turkey and face another 'no sweet foods' tyrannical diet. That won't work for you. We can apply to sugar much of the advice I gave you for cutting down painlessly on fats.

Make changes gradually
If you do take sugar in tea or coffee and want to cut down, do so by a very small amount at a time. In a few weeks you may well be able to give up altogether. I know many people who used to take drinks sweetened and who now find the taste awful if sugar is added by mistake.

Make swops in what you buy and what you cook
You can satisfy a sweet tooth in all kinds of ways to reduce your calorie intake.

Look down the lists that follow. On the left are some of the most popular sweet foods, the full-calorie kind. The centre column gives alternatives that contain less fat and/or sugar and fewer calories; in other words, if you substitute each item in the second column for one in the first column regularly or even some of the time, you'll be cutting calories. The right-hand column consists of even better swops – i.e., they are even lower in fat and/or sugar and calories.

1 ⟶	2 ⟶	3
Fruit pie (300)	☐ Fruit pie made using artificial sweetener and filo pastry (180)	☐ Baked apple filled with mixed dried fruit and honey (150)
Fruit crumble and custard (400)	☐ Banana and low-fat custard (180)	☐ Banana (80)
Gâteau (300)	☐ Fruit fool (200)	☐ Fresh fruit salad (150)
Luxury ice cream cornet e.g. Cornetto (200)	☐ Soft ice cone e.g. Mr Whippy (90)	☐ 75 ml (3 fl oz) Shape low-fat ice cream (58)
Strawberry trifle (300)	☐ Strawberry mousse (110)	☐ Strawberries with 1 teaspoon fructose and aerosol cream (80)
Cream cake (250)	☐ Teacake with low-fat spread and low-sugar jam (180)	☐ Iced fruit bun (120)
Danish pastry (350)	☐ Doughnut (225)	☐ 40 g (1½ oz) slice fruit malt loaf (110)
(Calories in brackets)		

You can decide for yourself whether an item in the first column is so appealing that it is one of the few sweet items you are going to have, at least now and then; whether you would be happy on most occasions with the middle alternatives; or whether you could sometimes choose some of the items in the last list. Tick all the items in both the second and third columns that you would be content to eat as alternatives to those in the first list, at least some of the time. Refer back to the list when you are stuck for ideas.

You can introduce further swops. In general it is always best to choose fresh fruit for a dessert or between-meal snack to satisfy your sweet tooth. Fresh fruit is low or fairly low in calories, virtually fat-free and contains vitamins and fibre. Next best is dried fruit (no added sugar) of all kinds. This contains lots of natural sugar so is very sweet, but has vitamins, minerals and plenty of fibre. It will keep you feeling full for longer. You could also consider having a handful of breakfast cereal such as Fruit 'n' Fibre or bran flakes, which are quite sweet but relatively 'good for you'. Lastly, diet yogurt or fromage frais (at around 50 calories each) are both low in fat and will satisfy that craving for the creamy taste that so many high-cal desserts give you.

ACTION

Think of some more swops of your own. Write your favourite desserts/sweet treats on the left here. In the centre column write down the names of types of food that are similar but contain less fat. Then, on the right, add an item from the above suggestions that you enjoy.

1 $\longrightarrow$	2 $\longrightarrow$	3
•	....	....
•	....	....
•	....	....
•	....	....
•	....	....

Here are two further suggestions. If you don't like artificial sweetener, use fructose (fruit sugar) instead of sucrose (table sugar). Fructose is twice as sweet as sugar, so you can halve quantities, and it's suitable for cooking. Because it isn't absorbed into the bloodstream as rapidly as sucrose, it will help prevent the low blood-sugar rebound that leaves many sweet-toothers feeling tired or faint after a binge on sweet food.

Don't forget, too, always to choose low-calorie versions of soft drinks such as cola, squash and lemonade. If you consume these types of drink in large quantities, it is best to replace them when you can with healthier drinks such as diluted fruit juice or mineral water.

*   *   *

'I'm a chocoholic'

Well, we had to get round to the subject of chocolate eventually, didn't we? Chocolate is nice, there is no denying that. And there is no reason why you have to give up the taste of chocolate even while you are slimming.

The reason I know this is that almost everybody eats chocolate yet very many of these people are not overweight. The way to tame your chocolate 'addiction', to make it something you can contain within a reasonable diet, is to look at the people who eat chocolate and aren't fat on it – and see what they are doing that you are not doing, and vice versa.

Keep a 'chocolate diary'

For a week, write down in your notepad every time you eat chocolate and alongside each entry describe briefly how you felt directly before you ate it – and what you think made you eat it.

Here are the most likely reasons you will have come up with:

'I was miserable/bored'   At times when you eat chocolate for comfort, turn to pages 125–30 for advice on dealing with those situations; then come back to this page.

'I was hungry'   One of the few times it isn't a good idea to eat chocolate is when you are hungry. That is because all the sugar in most chocolate products is absorbed quickly into the bloodstream (see above) and soon has you feeling hungry again. So eating high-fat, high-sugar foods like chocolate instead of a nutrient-high meal is a bad habit to get into.

If you often find yourself grabbing chocolate when you are hungry, it is important to plan ahead and ensure you have something other than chocolate ready at hand. Could you pop a sandwich or some filling fruit in your bag or pocket? Could you allow yourself more time to buy or prepare a proper snack when you are hungry? Why has chocolate frequently been your only answer to filling yourself up? Turn to pages 119–123 for more suggestions on how to eat 'on the run'.

'I was given it/it was just there'   If you're offered food you don't really want or need, be it chocolate or anything else, and you have a job saying no, then turn to pages 102–104 for more advice on dealing with that predicament.

'It's my birthday!'   Well, fine, eat your chocolate and enjoy it! No one is going to get fat on chocolate eaten once a year, or even on his/her birthday *and* at Christmas and Easter. It's daily chocolate bingeing you have to get under control. But, interestingly enough, most people who reduce their chocolate intake on a regular basis report that, when they *do* try to have a real choccie binge, they can't manage a quarter of the amount they used to. 'After half a box of my old favourites, I felt quite sick and had a really nasty cloying taste in my mouth. I had to clean my teeth!' said a friend of mine who has managed to beat the chocolate habit and indulged once after a few months' eating very little of it.

'I just love chocolate!'   You eat chocolate simply and purely because you love the taste. In that case, if you want to lose weight without giving up that pleasure, you can either:

1. *Settle for a reasonable chocolate allowance* – either a smaller amount on a daily basis or a larger amount on a weekly basis – be happy to lose weight at a slower rate than perhaps you might have done (see Step Four) and savour your chocolate, or:

2. *Learn to make 'chocolate swops'.* Not all chocolatey things are as high-calorie as others. If it's the taste you're after, you can get a satisfying one that involves only a quarter of the calories. I've drawn up a swop chart here to give you some ideas. All you do when you feel like having something out of the left-hand column is pick instead one of the things in the right-hand column. You'll find most of the items on the right will fit quite well into your pyramid-style diet, about which more in Step Four.

Swop this …	*for this …*
Mars Bar, standard (280)	Lo Bar (100)
Chocolate digestive biscuit (85)	Choc Chip Cookie (40)
Choc and nut Cornetto ice cream (210)	Choc ice (120)
Chocolate milk shake (300)	Ovaltine Options (40)
Slice choc fudge cake (300)	Individual choc cup cake (130)
Chocolate cheesecake (300)	Individual choc mousse (100)
Kit Kat (245)	Choc Chip Chewy Bar (120)
Profiteroles (300-400)	1 Dairy Cream Eclair (120)
Individual choc sponge (300)	Chocolate Puddi (115)

(Calories in brackets)

Also, don't forget that a little chocolate spread goes a long way and, on a slice of wholemeal bread, makes quite a nutritious meal. And another way to get a chocolatey taste on desserts – say, a bowl of fresh strawberries or some low-calorie vanilla ice cream – is to add a dash of chocolate sauce.

Cold turkey? If you're a lifelong chocolate addict, should you try to go cold turkey and give it up altogether, at one go? I think not.

REMEMBER!

Most slim people eat chocolate and manage to stay slim. That's because sometimes they take it, sometimes they leave it.

You've got to realise that, just because you like chocolate, you aren't a weak-willed, self-indulgent, hopeless case. Far from it. You're like everyone else: you *can* choose when to eat chocolate and enjoy it – and when not to. The rest of Step Three will be very helpful in getting that craving under control, but, in my experience, if people say they are giving up chocolate altogether, it only makes them want it all the more. There's no need! Remember, you don't need willpower to lose weight! You're not in an 'all or nothing' situation any more. You're not following a tyrannical diet. Managing chocolate may take time, but you'll do it.

*   *   *

'I don't enjoy healthy foods so how can I diet?'
'I don't like salads or many vegetables.'

What people who say they don't like 'health foods' – particularly salads and vegetables – in my experience really mean is one of the following:

'I don't like certain things that appear to me to come under the category "health foods"' (e.g., brown rice, beansprouts, grapefruit, figs).

'I dislike certain vegetables and salads because I associate them with unappetising offerings in the past' (e.g., watery, overboiled greens and limp lettuce salads).

'I haven't tried many of these foods but I don't think I would like them'.

None of these feelings, when you examine them closely, actually mean that you won't like eating in a slimmer, more healthy way *if* you accept that some of your old ideas and prejudices may be wrong.

Look at the chart that follows. There are four lists of food items. Go down each list and tick which box in the columns alongside applies to you for every food.

List One

	Like	Will eat	Haven't tried	Dislike at present
White bread	☐	☐	☐	☐
Brown bread	☐	☐	☐	☐
Wholemeal bread	☐	☐	☐	☐
Rye bread	☐	☐	☐	☐
Speciality breads (e.g., Ciabatta)	☐	☐	☐	☐
Pitta	☐	☐	☐	☐
Crispbread	☐	☐	☐	☐
Crustini sticks	☐	☐	☐	☐
Grissini sticks	☐	☐	☐	☐
Baked potatoes	☐	☐	☐	☐
Boiled potatoes	☐	☐	☐	☐
Mashed potatoes	☐	☐	☐	☐
Sweet potatoes	☐	☐	☐	☐
Baked beans	☐	☐	☐	☐
Butter beans	☐	☐	☐	☐
Red kidney beans	☐	☐	☐	☐
Black-eye beans	☐	☐	☐	☐
Chick peas	☐	☐	☐	☐
Green lentils	☐	☐	☐	☐
Home-made lentil soup	☐	☐	☐	☐
Weetabix	☐	☐	☐	☐
Porridge	☐	☐	☐	☐

	Like	Will eat	Haven't tried	Dislike at present
Bran flakes	☐	☐	☐	☐
Fruit 'n' Fibre	☐	☐	☐	☐
Spaghetti	☐	☐	☐	☐
Tagliatelle	☐	☐	☐	☐
Lasagne	☐	☐	☐	☐
Brown rice	☐	☐	☐	☐
Long-grain rice	☐	☐	☐	☐
Wild rice	☐	☐	☐	☐
Couscous	☐	☐	☐	☐
Bulgar wheat	☐	☐	☐	☐
Buckwheat	☐	☐	☐	☐
Pancakes	☐	☐	☐	☐
Polenta	☐	☐	☐	☐
Noodles	☐	☐	☐	☐

List Two

	Like	Will eat	Haven't tried	Dislike at present
Apple	☐	☐	☐	☐
Apricots, fresh	☐	☐	☐	☐
Apricots, dried	☐	☐	☐	☐
Banana	☐	☐	☐	☐
Blackcurrants	☐	☐	☐	☐
Currants, dried	☐	☐	☐	☐
Cherries	☐	☐	☐	☐
Dates, fresh	☐	☐	☐	☐
Dates, dried	☐	☐	☐	☐
Gooseberries	☐	☐	☐	☐
Grapefruit, pink	☐	☐	☐	☐

	Like	Will eat	Haven't tried	Dislike at present
Grapes	☐	☐	☐	☐
Kiwifruit	☐	☐	☐	☐
Mango	☐	☐	☐	☐
Melon, water	☐	☐	☐	☐
Melon, ogen	☐	☐	☐	☐
Nectarine	☐	☐	☐	☐
Orange	☐	☐	☐	☐
Peaches, fresh	☐	☐	☐	☐
Peaches, dried	☐	☐	☐	☐
Pears, fresh	☐	☐	☐	☐
Pears, dried	☐	☐	☐	☐
Prunes, Californian	☐	☐	☐	☐
Prunes, stoned	☐	☐	☐	☐
Raspberries	☐	☐	☐	☐
Rhubarb	☐	☐	☐	☐
Satsuma	☐	☐	☐	☐
Strawberries	☐	☐	☐	☐

List Three

	Like	Will eat	Haven't tried	Dislike at present
Artichoke, Jerusalem	☐	☐	☐	☐
Artichoke hearts	☐	☐	☐	☐
Asparagus	☐	☐	☐	☐
Aubergine	☐	☐	☐	☐
Avocado	☐	☐	☐	☐
Beans, broad	☐	☐	☐	☐
Beans, French	☐	☐	☐	☐
Beans, runner	☐	☐	☐	☐

	Like	Will eat	Haven't tried	Dislike at present
Beansprouts	☐	☐	☐	☐
Beetroot	☐	☐	☐	☐
Broccoli	☐	☐	☐	☐
Brussels sprouts	☐	☐	☐	☐
Cabbage, green	☐	☐	☐	☐
Cabbage, red	☐	☐	☐	☐
Cabbage, white	☐	☐	☐	☐
Carrots	☐	☐	☐	☐
Cauliflower	☐	☐	☐	☐
Celery	☐	☐	☐	☐
Chinese leaves	☐	☐	☐	☐
Corn on the cob	☐	☐	☐	☐
Courgettes	☐	☐	☐	☐
Cucumber	☐	☐	☐	☐
Leek	☐	☐	☐	☐
Lettuce	☐	☐	☐	☐
Mushrooms	☐	☐	☐	☐
Onion, Spanish	☐	☐	☐	☐
Onion, spring	☐	☐	☐	☐
Onion, red	☐	☐	☐	☐
Parsnip	☐	☐	☐	☐
Peas, fresh	☐	☐	☐	☐
Peas, frozen	☐	☐	☐	☐
Pepper, green	☐	☐	☐	☐
Pepper, red	☐	☐	☐	☐
Spinach, fresh	☐	☐	☐	☐

	Like	Will eat	Haven't tried	Dislike at present
Swede	☐	☐	☐	☐
Sweetcorn	☐	☐	☐	☐
Tomato	☐	☐	☐	☐
Tomato, cherry	☐	☐	☐	☐
Watercress	☐	☐	☐	☐

List Four

	Like	Will eat	Haven't tried	Dislike at present
Low-fat soft cheese	☐	☐	☐	☐
Diet cottage cheese	☐	☐	☐	☐
Cod	☐	☐	☐	☐
Monkfish	☐	☐	☐	☐
Brill	☐	☐	☐	☐
Lemon sole	☐	☐	☐	☐
Trout, brown	☐	☐	☐	☐
Trout, rainbow	☐	☐	☐	☐
Tuna in brine	☐	☐	☐	☐
Salmon, fresh	☐	☐	☐	☐
Crabmeat	☐	☐	☐	☐
Mussels	☐	☐	☐	☐
Prawns	☐	☐	☐	☐
Scallops	☐	☐	☐	☐
Squid	☐	☐	☐	☐
Turkey	☐	☐	☐	☐
Venison	☐	☐	☐	☐
Quorn	☐	☐	☐	☐
Tofu	☐	☐	☐	☐
TVP mince	☐	☐	☐	☐

	Like	Will eat	Haven't tried	Dislike at present
Fromage frais, natural	☐	☐	☐	☐
Natural low-fat Bio yogurt	☐	☐	☐	☐
Natural whole-milk yogurt	☐	☐	☐	☐

This isn't intended to be a comprehensive list of all available 'healthy' foods, by the way, but it is a fair cross section.

Now look back through your ticks.

If you have some ticks in each list under the 'Like' or 'Will eat' headings, then you have a sound basis for forming a slimmer, healthier diet without doing much more. These are the foods that you can eat and enjoy without any problems and no more adjustments. Make the most of them!

If you have ticks under the 'Haven't tried' heading, well, great. Here is a marvellous opportunity for you to discover some new foods and make your slimming and weight maintenance diet more interesting. One of the keys to taking control of your diet and your figure successfully is the willingness to try some new things, and never to condemn anything until you have tried it. (See below for ways to incorporate new foods into your diet.)

If you have ticks under the 'Dislike at present' heading, don't be disheartened. Remember, you don't *have* to eat any of these foods (assuming you haven't ticked the 'dislike' box for absolutely everything!). But do keep an open mind while you read on to the end of page 98. By trying some of the ideas here you may find that, in fact, you can turn a 'dislike' food into a 'like' food.

REMEMBER!

You don't have to make sweeping changes, but don't be afraid to experiment. Research shows that humans are instinctively suspicious of brand-new foods (a throwback to those long-ago days when eating a wrong food – say, a poisonous berry – could kill you, so it paid to be wary) but also have a strong taste for adventure and a fairly low boredom threshold.

Translated into your diet, that means that the two best ways to incorporate new foods into it are by (a) adding them to something familiar – e.g., adding lentils to a cottage pie, or a few fresh beansprouts to your favourite stir-fry, or (b) preparing them in a familiar way. For instance, suppose you are going to try the low-fat protein food Quorn, or tofu. There is more chance you will enjoy it if, instead of following a totally new recipe to cook it, you use it in a familiar recipe, such as a pie where you would normally use chicken. This is an excellent tip for introducing children to new foods, too.

Experimenting also means using familiar foods in different ways. This is one of the keys to swopping painlessly from an old-fashioned British diet to a new-style pyramid diet. If you love beef, for instance, find new recipes that require smaller quantities of beef – e.g., beef and vegetable soup, or certain Chinese dishes.

The modern 'composite-style' dishes are the perfect vehicle for the pyramid-style approach. Try all the time to think not of the 'meat with a veg' type of meal, but the kind in which all the ingredients are mixed. Pastas and grains of all kinds, including rice, noodles and other of the fairly bland complex carbohydrate foods, can be transformed when they become part of an exotic Mediterranean, Far or Middle Eastern or other ethnic dish. (For ideas on this type of cooking, see recipe section.)

It's also time to begin experimenting with condiments. How many of the following have you tried?

☐	Mushroom sauce	☐	Cajun seasoning
☐	Oyster sauce	☐	Five-spice seasoning
☐	Soya sauce	☐	Home-made curry blends
☐	Hot chilli sauce	☐	Saffron
☐	Anchovy essence	☐	Coconut milk

☐ Passata ☐ Basil
☐ Balsamic vinegar ☐ Fresh chillies
☐ Wine vinegar ☐ Yellow-bean sauce
☐ Whole-grain mustard ☐ Lemon grass
☐ Lime juice ☐ Oregano

These are just a few of the fabulous flavourings now available nationwide to help make our cooking exciting and tasty.

This is where the local delicatessens, the health-food shops and, especially, the supermarkets really come up trumps. They are an Aladdin's cave of fabulous ingredients – mostly inexpensive, often complete with recipes, or at least usage suggestions, attached – which can help transform your diet in the most subtle ways. You don't *need* fat to make food interesting these days. And you need never, ever, again say healthy food is boring if you are prepared to keep an open mind and make the most of what's available from your local food shops.

REMEMBER!

It's up to you how you choose and what you cook. (If it isn't, turn to sections 2 and 3 for more advice.) Let's suppose that you are a 'vegetable hater' or a 'salad hater'. Our mums and grandparents have a lot to answer for when it comes to instilling in the nation a dislike of all green vegetables! For some reason, the British have never been all that hot at preparing and cooking vegetables, which can and should be delicious in all their varieties. Instead, they have all too often been served up as a tasteless, tough and/or soggy mess.

Don't ignore the vegetable counters any longer just because of a long-standing prejudice. Now you can buy fantastic vegetables from all over the world (for which, again, we must thank the modern 'global village' food industry and your local supermarket) in dozens of varieties. Baby vegetables ranging from baby cauliflower to baby aubergines are a wonderful choice, for instance.

And, once you've chosen, think of all the different ways they can be used. You can roast all kinds, as well as stir-fry, steam, braise, purée, and use them in thousands of different recipes. This again is the new-style pyramid way of eating, with composite dishes rather than separate little mounds on your plate (not that there's anything wrong with that occasionally).

Salads, too, don't need to be of the limp, 'watery lettuce' and 'tasteless tomato' variety. Just stop and have a good look at the salad counters. These foods may not be advertised on TV or in the magazines, but they should be! Sample some new salad ingredients and try them in different ways – then tell me you don't like salad! Experiment with rice salads, pasta salads, mixed salads including fruits, salads with pulses such as flageolet beans, salads with herbs, salads with spiced dressings. It is only your imagination stopping you from enjoying salads! There are some recommendations for you further on in this book – and I do urge you also to go to the library or bookshop and check out some modern cookery books for more ideas.

ACTION

Before we leave this 'I don't like healthy food' discussion, here's one last test for you.

Enlist a friend to help you. Invite him or her round for supper or lunch and serve a salad or soup starter, a main-course dish and a dessert, all from the recipes that appear later in this book, following all the methods exactly and using all the lower-fat, healthy ingredients. Don't say anything about the meal to your friend. When you have finished eating, ask if (s)he noticed anything unusual. The answer is bound to be 'no'. Then, and only then, you can tell your friend that everything (s)he ate had only about half the calories and fat of 'normal' versions!

*   *   *

*'When I see available food, I eat it
even if I'm not hungry.'*
*'Once I open a pack of something,
I can't stop until it's empty.'*
'I always eat up everything I'm given.'

If you often find yourself saying these things or feeling this way, you are an 'automatic eater', downing many unnecessary calories a day on 'automatic pilot'. Overcoming this habit alone may well be enough to help you lose weight with little need to cut the calories in other ways. And it's not difficult. Putting food into your mouth when you're not hungry – just thoughtless – is a habit. It may be a long-standing habit, but it is one you can control. Remember, food is an inanimate object with no mind of its own. *You* have a mind of your own. You can learn to say 'no'.

You can defeat old habits most easily by adopting this approach:

1. Learn to *focus* on what you are doing.
2. *Decide* whether what you are putting in your mouth is what you really want.
3. *Say 'no'* to yourself (and others if necessary) by the easiest possible means available. Use 'props' or a 'step-by-step' approach if appropriate.

More of this 'focus-decide-say no' system in a minute, but first let's find out how often you eat on 'automatic pilot'.

Keep a record of everything you eat during the course of today or tomorrow. Write it down in the chart on the next page and fill out the 'reason' column. Leave the solution column blank for the time being.

To help you, overleaf is an example of how one mother might account for some of her 'automatic pilot eating' on a typical day.

We will return to your list at the end of the discussion and you can fill in your own solutions.

Food eaten	Time	Reason	Solution
Half a pack crunchy nut biscuits	9 a.m.	Opened pack for son's lunch-box. Ate without thinking	Will try to concentrate on what I'm doing in future
Fish portion in batter, fried	6.30 p.m.	Cooked it for child who said he wanted two and ate only one	Cook less in future – he often can't eat up all his food
Pack of mini choc eggs	8 p.m.	Fancied something sweet while watching TV. Didn't realise I'd eaten whole pack	Have a piece of fruit instead, or, put out 'allowed' amount of treat before I sit down

Your own diary

Food eaten	Time	Reason	Solution

Shopping and food planning

If you shop for food regularly and mostly eat at home, you should tackle 'automatic eating' at its root cause – in the supermarket. What you eat begins with what you buy. What you don't have in the house you can't just help yourself to; in other words, you can't eat without some effort (e.g., you have to go out again and buy it).

Tick the statements that apply to you:

☐ I rarely or never write a shopping list

☐ I go shopping when hungry

☐ I go into a shop with little idea of what I'm going to buy

☐ I buy things with little idea of who is going to eat them, or when

☐ I buy items that don't co-ordinate with each other or that will all be at their 'eat by' date together

☐ I am easily swayed by multi-pack savings and special offers or by my children asking for things they see

If you ticked several of these statements, you have been allowing the supermarket or store to dominate you. You will save money – and many calories – by being a more organised shopper and food planner.

You can take control and *use* the many benefits of the modern shops and supermarkets to help you. It requires less time to be organised than disorganised, but it does take some practice. Here are the main tips that will help you shop to avoid mindless eating later at home.

● Plan, as far ahead as possible, what you intend to eat. If you can plan for a week at a time, so much the better. Write down all the meals you will have and then convert this into a shopping list including amounts. Organise your list into 'like groups' – e.g., all the fruits together, all the veg, all the dairy produce, and so on. That way, impulse buying is less likely to grip you.

- If you are a 'nibbler', include on the list several low- or fairly low-fat and calorie items which will, at least at first, replace some of the higher-fat, higher-cal things you've been used to nibbling.

- Before you go shopping, repeat to yourself: 'Yes, I *can* stick to the list!'

- Shop soon after you have eaten. It is well known that if you shop when hungry you buy more, especially of the 'instant energy', ready-made foods like biscuits and chocolate bars. If possible, shop when you are in a positive and happy frame of mind.

- Shop infrequently. The list system should make sure you don't have to keep dashing to the shop for things you forgot. Today, with freezers, fridges and so many long-life products available, you should be able to organise yourself around a weekly shopping trip. Most fruit and vegetables keep well for a week, especially if you pick them under-ripe and store them cool.

- Tempted by a special offer or multi-pack even so? Try to visualise who will eat it and when. Avoid big packs of anything if you don't have a big family. Remember, we live in a society of plenty. We eat more than we need because we take home in our shopping bags more than we needed to buy.

Eating food because it's there

How many of these do you do? *Tick the statements that apply to you:*

☐ I take food that's offered me without even considering whether or not I want it (e.g., canapés at a drinks party – or, indeed, another drink at a drinks party)

☐ I keep dipping my hand into the peanuts or crisps at a bar or party or into the bag of sweets at home, until they are all gone

☐ I eat the roll and butter at a restaurant or the free mints afterwards

☐ I always eat a pudding after the main course because that is what I have always done

☐ I go to the café at lunchtime to buy a sandwich and I come out with a Danish pastry too, because the tray was right in front of my eyes

These are classic cases of 'automatic pilot' action, which we can defeat by returning to the three-step approach:

(1) Focus. (2) Decide. (3) Say 'no'.

Here are some examples of that system at work.

✱ **BEAT** automatically accepting food that's offered.
Focus on what you are doing. (I am about to accept food because it is being offered, literally, on a plate.)
Decide. (Do I really need it? If I have a few of these, how will I feel? I only ate an hour or two ago. I'm going to say 'no'.)
Say 'no' in the easiest possible way. (If a waiter is offering, it is no problem just to shake your head. If it's a friend, smile and say: 'I've just had one, thanks!')

✱ **BEAT** the urge to dip your hand in the peanut tray (or whatever).
Focus on what you are doing. (This takes practice but learn to be aware of your hand moving to your mouth each time.)
Decide. (No, this is ridiculous, I've had enough of these nuts/crisps/sweets, so why am I eating them?)
Say 'no', using props (ask barman to take crisps away/move them down the bar yourself/get up and replace the taste with something else, e.g., a mint if you've been eating savouries).

If the 'nibble food' is in the home, ask yourself: *Why is it in the home?* Have you been planning and shopping wisely?

✱ **BEAT** the urge to eat all the extras during your restaurant meal. How easy it is to get through the bread basket while you decide what you are going to choose from the menu!
Focus. (I am getting through an awful lot of this bread and butter.)
Decide. (I am hungry but if I eat much of this it will spoil my appetite for the food I really want.)
Say 'no'. (Move basket to another table/ask waiter to take it away/get up and visit loo/take a drink of water.)

✱ **BEAT** 'because I always have eaten desserts.'
Focus. (I'm eating this because I've been doing so for years.)
Decide. (I expect it's all these sweet things when I'm full that help to make me fat. I'd like to try to cut them down or out somehow.)
Say 'no'. (Perhaps use the step-by-step technique. First take smaller portions; then change to a lighter dessert – e.g., a yogurt – then to a piece of fresh fruit.)

✱ **BEAT** the urge to buy extra when you go to the takeaway.
Focus. (I've come here for a sandwich but I can see those pretty pastries there. However, I know they have been put there just to tempt people like me.)
Decide. (I had no intention of buying one before I came in, so why should I change my mind?)
Say 'no'. (Use props to bolster your resolve. Find a different sandwich shop where they don't display the sweet foods under your nose. Or ask a colleague if (s)he'll buy your sandwich for you. Or take your own lunch to work.)

Cleaning the plate

Many people continue to eat long after they feel full up simply because there is still food on their plate. Other people will polish off leftovers on a similar principle, usually without consciously thinking about it. But I believe that for the young much of this attitude is an inherited one. The idea that it was a dreadful waste to leave anything on the plate began during the food-lean war years. Older readers may themselves remember those years.

Our next discussion about the difference between hunger and appetite will help solve this problem but you should also adopt the three-stage approach.

Focus: learn to concentrate on your eating and recognise the point at which you feel full rather than the point at which the plate is clean.

Decide: 'I have had enough to satisfy my hunger. If I have any more I will be eating unnecessary calories.'

Say 'no': stop eating. Remove the plate. Use props. If you prepared the food, obviously the answer is to put less on your plate. If you are a guest, ask the preparer to serve you a smaller portion. Should there habitually be a lot of food wastage in your house, you need to rethink at the planning and shopping stage and prepare a smaller amount of food for meals. Habitually buying and preparing too much food is a waste of money and resources – and eating it isn't the answer.

Eating while watching TV

I bet that more calories are consumed unnecessarily while people watch television than in any other way! It is so easy to sit and munch your way through a monster bag of crisps or chocolates or biscuits while your mind is on the TV. Or you may even do the same while reading a book or magazine. This really is 'mindless eating'. Then the TV commercials make matters worse: even if you hadn't been snacking, a tempting ad for some food snack or other comes on ... and up you get and find something to eat.

To help beat 'TV eating', follow the three-stage method.

Focus: train yourself to be aware that you are putting something in your mouth.
Decide: are you really hungry? Why are you eating?
Say 'no': use props.

- Find something else to do while watching TV – e.g., sew, knit; have a paper ready to occupy you during the boring bits.
- Get up and do something else. One of the reasons we eat while watching TV is that we're bored. If you're bored, why are you watching? Is there really nothing else you would like to do?
- If you have a remote control, switch channels while the commercials are on.
- Chew calorie-free gum while you adapt to not snacking in front of the TV.
- If you're not strong enough to give up snacking altogether, switch from crisps/chocolates/biscuits to, say, Grissini (Italian bread sticks) or grapes.
- Lastly, remember that what you didn't buy you can't eat, so remove temptation by being a wiser shopper.

Saying no and meaning it

Saying 'no' isn't easy at first, especially if you've usually given in. But you *can* overcome this tendency. At first, as you've seen, you can get plenty of help from 'props' of various kinds. Then, of course, because new habits soon become familiar old habits, the sooner you can grab hold of a new habit and make it your own, the easier it becomes. Eventually it becomes an old habit that is easy to live with.

It may help you to refuse more easily if you have an outside motivation that helps you to feel better about yourself every time you do it successfully.

The best idea of all is to start a fund box. Every time you manage to say 'no' to a food you didn't need and didn't really want, put a set amount of money in the fund box (you decide how much, but don't make it too much or you won't do it). At the end of every month, empty the box and give half of the proceeds to your favourite charity – in the circumstances, I would suggest famine relief(!) but it is up to you – and put the other half towards a non-food treat for yourself.

RETURN TO THE DIARY

Now let's go back to that one-day's food diary you began on page 100. Look through all the things you ate that day. How many of these did you eat mindlessly, 'on automatic pilot'?

Now, bearing in mind all you have learnt in this discussion, try to think of your own solution for each of those items. Use the **Focus – Decide – Say 'no'** system, thinking of props or step-by-step techniques as necessary. I can help you solve your food problems, but you can help yourself, too!

*   *   *

'I can't bear the idea of feeling hungry.'
'Food is one of my few pleasures in life.'

You want to be slim but you don't want to deprive yourself, either through having to feel hungry or by having to give up the sheer pleasure that eating can bring. That's natural – and you needn't.

HUNGRY AGAIN?

If you have been overeating for a long time, you may have lost touch with your body's own ability to tell you when you are hungry. The deeply ingrained fear of hunger was, long ago, a perfectly reasonable one: after all, then man truly didn't know when or from where his next meal was coming. But the fear of hunger that permanently keeps us eating just that little bit *more* is one of the main reasons we get fat.

Many overweight people have *never* felt genuinely hungry in their lives. So the very thought of being made to feel hungry on a diet is enough to put them in a panic.

But the point is that you don't *have* to feel permanently ravenous while you are slimming. (Some diets may have made you feel that way in the past but they were wrong.) What you *should* do is feel hungry – and then satisfy that hunger by eating something. You really mustn't feel hungry and then not eat anything. In fact, one of the most important messages in *Slim for Life* is: *always eat something if you feel hungry*. If you can get back to eating in a way that obeys your hunger instincts – to eat when you are hungry and eat nothing when you're not, you will be well on the way to conquering your weight problem for good.

So what you need to do is relearn the difference between real hunger and 'false hunger'. Let's look at that now.

Real hunger
How to tell if you are hungry:

- You may be able to hear and feel rumblings in your tummy. That is your stomach reminding you that it would like something to eat.
- You may have 'hunger pangs' – a gnawing or empty feeling higher up in your stomach.
- You will probably not have eaten for at least two or three hours.
- You may have taken some recent prolonged exercise – e.g., a morning's walk.

A real appetite is what you get when you are genuinely hungry. People's appetite varies from day to day and also, in the case of women, from week to week during the menstrual cycle. And, of course, it varies according to how much work (activity) your body has been doing.

The *Slim for Life* programme in Step Four helps you to avoid long periods of hunger (which you may have suffered in the past on other diets) in these ways:

- You learn your hungry times of day and plan your slimming campaign to take account of them.
- You learn your hungry times of the month/year and, again, plan accordingly.
- You eat more if you are active.
- You are guided to a suitable food intake that takes account of your own metabolic needs.
- You eat plenty of the types of food that 'release energy slowly' and which stop you from feeling hungry again quickly after a meal.
- You avoid the type of sweet foods that provoke wildly fluctuating blood-sugar levels and 'rebound hunger'.
- You may eat as frequently as you like so you need never *fear* hunger.

False hunger

Many of us often feel false hunger and overweight people tend to feel it more frequently than slim people. This way they are 'conned' into eating when they don't need to. Here are the main 'false hunger' situations and how to deal with them:

Taste experience   How often have you reckoned yourself full to the brim after the main course of a meal but suddenly felt able to eat again when the dessert trolley came round? Your poor old flagging appetite has been stimulated by the thought of trying a new taste, a new texture, after what has gone before. Making this choice occasionally – and allowing for it – won't harm you, but if you habitually override your natural instinct that says 'I'm full' and continue to 'eat for taste' you will have problems. Deal with this step by step. You're faced with a dessert trolley, say. You then have three courses of action to choose from: you can opt for a plate of fresh fruit and 'steal' a bit of what you fancy from your partner's plate; you can ask for a half portion; or you can take the decision to say 'no' and discover the pleasure that springs from knowing you can control false hunger just as well as a slim person can.

Habit hunger   If you always eat at fixed times, whether or not you are hungry, and then are annoyed to find yourself hungry at an hour when you don't normally eat, you are too much of a slave to the clock. It is perhaps convenient to eat at set times but it isn't particularly natural. If you can get more in tune with your natural 'body clock' it will help you to stay slim.

For example, many people I know don't feel hungry at breakfast time but, because it is traditional, they sit down to a breakfast. By mid-morning they do feel hungry, so they eat something else. Why not skip the breakfast and make mid-morning the 'breakfast' time to eat when you will really enjoy doing so? Another example: many people eat their evening meal at around 6 p.m. when they get home from work and a lot of them will be starving by 9 p.m. Why not have the evening meal a little later? Take a look at your meal times and see whether they really do fit in with your body needs.

Trigger foods   Perhaps you're familiar with this syndrome: you eat a meal, then, an hour later, wander down the street past the baker's and find yourself desperate for a cream doughnut. This is a 'trigger food'. The foods that are most likely to trigger your appetite are fresh bread and other bakery items, cheese, and chocolate. The best ploy here is avoidance tactics – e.g., walk down a different street so you don't have to pass the baker's. If it isn't possible to steer clear, you have to decide whether instead you will allow yourself that food in amounts controlled by you (remember, food is an inanimate object; *you* are the boss), or else replace the 'trigger food' with something less calorific and less appealing to you – e.g., Edam instead of your favourite Stilton cheese, a crusty wholemeal roll instead of a croissant. (For chocolate suggestions, see page 88.)

ACTION

1. Write down, on the chart below, everything you eat for a day, as soon as you've eaten it if possible. Then decide which of the 'hungers' made you eat it. (Some items you may have eaten for other reasons dealt with in other parts of this section, in which case ignore them.)

Time	Food eaten	Reason			
		Genuine hunger	Taste	Habit	Trigger

2. Now try going for a whole day waiting until you feel genuine hunger before you eat and keep a record here.

Time	Food eaten

When you feel hungry, eat a 'pyramid-type' meal – a complex carbohydrate with a little low-fat protein and some vegetables and fruit. Eat slowly and chew thoroughly. Carry on eating until you feel full, then stop.

Try to do this every day – and bear in mind what you have already learnt in this section: to plan ahead, to exercise reasonable portion control and to keep in mind that *you* are in control.

You are learning to take heed of your own hunger patterns and body needs. Don't let false hunger override those needs; then you really will be on the way to permanent slimness!

Food as pleasure

Ever since the beginning of mankind, we humans have found eating to be a pleasure. For most of us, it is a nice thing to do and that's why we offer food to people we like; why we enjoy sharing a meal with friends; and why special occasions are celebrated with special food. From the huge banquets of the rich in the Middle Ages through to the small dinner parties of the 1990s, food equals the good life.

These days, we tend to celebrate more frequently, albeit on a less grand scale. Food, for most of us, is always available. Virtually anyone who can afford it is able to rustle up a mini-feast for friends or find a handy restaurant or bar.

And just as our tastebuds lead us to try a wide variety of foods, so they lead us to try a wide variety of restaurants, cafés, bistros and bars, and to feel delighted when we are invited to someone's home for a meal.

Should you be lucky enough to lead an active social life revolving around food and drink, you will be reluctant to give it up. Indeed, you don't need to socialise to enjoy eating; I know several people leading solitary lives who take delight in their food.

However, I have to assume that, if you're reading this book, your love of food has made you fat. You don't have to give up the pleasure of eating, but what you do have to do is take on board the practical advice you are finding on these pages. You need to replace your 'old-style' eating with 'new-style' eating and – if you recall the discussion on fat and how to reduce it without losing taste, and on how to enjoy the 'healthy' foods by using a variety of 'new' ingredients and your own imagination – I think you will agree that it is only your own reluctance that is stopping you from trying the new way now. Inviting friends round won't pose a problem (as the experiment on page 98 showed). Eating out isn't a predicament if you put into practice the cures for 'automatic pilot' eating (see page 99) and bear in mind the 'swops' principles. See, too, the large eating-out section in Step Four.

If it is the social whirl, rather than the actual eating, that particularly attracts you, don't forget that you can control what you eat virtually anywhere. In a restaurant, say, you can choose to skip the starter or dessert. You could even choose to meet your friends somewhere other than an eating place for a change. If you have a problem exercising enough assertiveness in this respect, read on to section 3, where you will learn how to cope with other people while you slim.

You don't have to stop enjoying food when you slim, you simply enjoy it in a slightly different way. Remember that if you can kill the guilt, which is what *Slim for Life* is helping you to do, you will enjoy your eating even more.

SECTION 2:

Handling the Lifestyle Factors

Are the circumstances in your life that seem to lead you to overeat *really* things you can do nothing about, or can you find ways to alter them? You can alter more than you imagine. And you can learn to alter your reaction to the things you really can't change. That's what section 2 is all about: controlling those 'circumstances beyond your control'.

> *'There is so much to do each day that I feel guilty if I spend time on myself, working out a diet, and so on.'*
>
> *'I tear round all the time and I just grab what food and drink is available.'*

It's better to be busy than bored, but if any of the above comments echo your own, you need to learn to give your needs priority at least some of the time in your life. Many people – particularly busy women with families and, often, careers too – feel there really is no 'spare' time to spend on themselves. Look down the list here. Which of the following things do you find time to do?

Tick the relevant boxes.

☐ Vacuum carpets   ☐ Wash car
☐ Iron clothes   ☐ Check oil and water in car

☐ Plant out windowboxes   ☐ Mow lawn

☐ Watch TV news   ☐ Clean oven

☐ Groom pet

If you ticked *any* of the above, you have time to spend on yourself. Why, for example, is your home or your car more important than your own body in the scheme of things? They obviously aren't, but you act as if they are. The fact is that within a busy life you make time for the things you consider most important. *You are important* and your body is important. To be slim and fit is to be healthier. We know that our car works better when it is regularly checked and serviced – and so do we. The car you can dispense with if it goes wrong, but you can't buy yourself a new body.

Also, making time for yourself helps your self-esteem. So get your priorities right and never feel guilty about from time to time doing things for *you* instead of for the house, the car, the family pet – even for the kids, the husband or wife, the boss or the best friend. Making time for yourself is your absolute right.

Time management

Some people manage their time much better than others and therefore succeed in packing a lot more into a day. If it seems to you that you're busy all the time, it would be a worthwhile exercise to do your own 'time and motion' study to see whether or not you are in fact wasting time.

- Do you frequently leave tasks half finished and come back to them later or another day?
- Do you pop out to the shops for just one item, then find yourself returning for another item later?
- Do you wake up in the morning without a clear idea of how you intend to spend the day?

If your answer is 'yes' to any of these questions, you could do with better time management. For this you need to learn about **focusing, planning** and **organisation.**

Focusing   This means spending time on thinking carefully about what you want to achieve, however big or little your objectives. If you don't think about what you want, you only ever find out what you want – and get what you want – by accident. You need to spend a little time every day on short-term aims and a little time every week on long-term aims.

Short-term aims are best thought about before you go to sleep at night. They could be anything from: 'I must wash my hair in the morning' or 'I must buy that new recipe book that my friend recommended' to: 'I must check out my store cupboard for things I need to start my new slimming campaign and also write a list of things I have to buy'.

Long-term aims are anything from: 'I must pick up some brochures from the travel agency and start planning my holiday' to: 'I must do some research and take notes before drawing up plans for redesigning the garden'.

To learn to focus on your body needs, it helps to ask yourself: 'How long since I … ?' This might be: 'How long since I last had a haircut?' 'How long since I last weighed myself?' 'How long since I last prepared a meal that I really wanted?'

Planning   This means deciding roughly what is feasible and what isn't – e.g., 'Can I cook that delicious-sounding low-fat recipe tonight or shall I think of something quicker?' or 'I'm not going to have time to see my friend tomorrow but I'll ring to arrange a get-together on Friday instead'.

Organisation   This means doing in the most sensible way what you have focused on and planned. It means writing lists in order of importance for the short-term aims; it means planning a schedule for each day as closely as you can (obviously life gets too regimented if you always live by a rigid agenda, but if time is short it really helps to have one).

The sad truth is that if you don't focus, plan and organise, then you will end up wasting time – your own time – and life – your own life.

If you've not been used to organising your life this way and then you do – again, it takes practice – you will be delighted to find that you do have a lot more time than you thought, time you can spend on recognising your body needs, getting slim and fit.

Priorities

If you already organise your life that way and you still don't make time for your body, you should now consider your priorities. Something has to go! So for two days write in your notebook everything you do, as you do it, jotting down alongside the time spent on each. After the two days are up, scrutinise the list and decide which of the things you did were least important. You may discover that you spend a lot of time being 'put upon' by others – running errands, being an agony aunt, helping out at charity events, for instance.

At this point you have to remind yourself that sometimes it is perfectly all right to say 'no' – not just to food, but to people. This is hard at first, especially if like many overweight people you suffer low self-esteem, which tends to make you want to please others. Two-thirds of the remedy is to learn to say 'no' in a nice but firm way. The other third is simply practice. Here are some examples of the way to refuse that should become part of your vocabulary.

- 'I'm so sorry, I can't fit that in today but I could probably manage it next week.'
- 'I would have loved you to come round now but I'm afraid I'm just going out of the door for an appointment.' (To the friend who cries on your shoulder at least once a day and has phoned you *again*.)
- 'I'll look in my diary … No, I'm so sorry, I'm already busy on that night.'
- 'I'm sorry, I can't help run that event – there is an important family anniversary on that day.'

● 'I would have loved to organise the charity sale this year but
  we're planning to go away on holiday during August.' (You
  can always change your mind about the holiday later!)

Don't feel guilty. Your time is precious too, and after a while
people will recognise this fact and will stop trying to overbur-
den you, so the problem of having to say 'no' will recede naturally. There's no need to turn everything and everyone down;
just do so now and then, and give yourself the time you need.

Have another look at your two-day diary. Are there tasks you
could have delegated to someone else (e.g., a child, partner,
home help, secretary, or other employee)? Most busy people
take on things someone else should or could be doing.

Lastly, are there things in the diary that you took too long
over because of habit? Could you speed up the handling of
some tasks where the end-result doesn't need to be first rate?

If you really and truly can't gain any time, accept the fact
that, long-term, your lifestyle needs to alter to give you more
relaxation. Make *that* one of your long-term aims.

Using the time you gain
Here are some suggestions for ways to use your new-found time
regularly and enjoyably:

Body time   Soak in the bath or take an invigorating shower;
do a manicure/pedicure; wash and style hair; have a massage;
do make time for some sport or a walk; have a makeover.

Food time   Plan some new low-fat menus; try out a specific
new recipe; eat your meal slowly and without interruptions;
shop for and prepare your food without feeling rushed or pres-
sured.

Mind time   Learn something new (from TV, book, radio,
class); listen to music; read something for pleasure; write something for pleasure (e.g., poem, letter, short story, diary).

Each night before you go to sleep, focus on what you want to do the next day. Aim to include at least one body thing, one food thing and one mind thing that you will really enjoy.

Remind yourself that eating a slimming, healthy diet doesn't in the long term take any longer than eating a fattening, unhealthy diet. At first it may take time to learn new habits, but not for long.

And, lastly, remember: it's *your* life. Enjoy it!

*   *   *

'*I travel a lot so I eat in pubs and snack bars.*'

'*As other people do the food shopping, I have no control.*'

'*I'm a student living in a bedsit with few cooking facilities, so how can I watch what I eat?*'

If you face any of these or similar situations where you seem to have little control over your meals, you have to ask yourself two questions:

- What can I reasonably expect to change about that situation?
- If I can't change the situation, how can I look at it differently?

First, you should for three days keep a food diary in your notebook. Draw up a chart of columns under these headings: *Day, Time, Food, Place, Source, Reason, Alternatives.* Fill in all the columns except the last one.

For instance, a student in a bedsit might have a day's diary like the one overleaf.

DAY: Monday

Time	Food	Place
8.30 a.m.	2 choc digestive biscuits	Room
11.00 a.m.	Choc bar	College
1.00 p.m.	Egg mayonnaise salad & roll/butter	College café
2.00 p.m.	Apple tart & ice cream	College café
5.00 p.m.	Crisps	College
6.00 p.m.	2 glasses cider	Pub
8.30 p.m.	Takeaway pizza	Room
11.00 p.m.	2 choc digestive biscuits	Room

Her lodging facilities include shared use of a fridge with a small freezer compartment and shared use of a basic cooker and toaster. There is a minimarket nearby which is quite expensive and a thrift store near college. 'I don't want to spend time doing much cooking. I'm not very good anyway,' she says. 'Life is so busy but I do want to slim.' The student plans her work schedule, so why not her eating schedule?

By planning ahead she could have improved her day's eating a lot. She could:

- Make a list of healthier things she likes to eat that can be stored in her room or the shared fridge: long-life juices, individual yogurts and fromage frais; under-ripe fruits in season; small sliced wholemeal loaf (could freeze half of it); low-fat spread; cans of tuna in brine; baked beans; Marmite; pure fruit spread; rye crispbreads; breakfast cereal; eggs; dried pasta; bottled tomato sauce; a tub low-fat soft cheese; a few tomatoes.

Source	Reason	Alternatives
Minimarket	Quick	
Vending machine	Quick: nothing else available	
College café	Lunchtime; salad is slimming	
College café	Still sitting talking, felt hungry	
Vending machine	Hungry	
Pub	Social	
Takeaway	Supper	
Minimarket	Bedtime	

- Shop for these once a week or fortnight in the thrift store.
- Have each day an easy breakfast such as cereal and long-life skimmed milk, or fromage frais and fruit.
- Take a piece of fruit for mid-morning.
- Have a college lunch (e.g., the egg salad without a dressing or with just a little mayonnaise). Ask for low-fat spread or soft margarine – which spreads thinner than butter – on the roll. Take a banana for dessert in case still hungry.
- Allow for an afternoon bag of crisps.
- Try a low-calorie drink in the pub sometimes.
- Allow for a takeaway (pizza isn't too bad) one or two nights a week, but try to have an easily prepared meal at home sometimes – e.g., pasta boiled and topped with ready-made tomato sauce; beans on toast; tomato salad with low-fat cheese; or tuna plus bread.
- For hungry-time snacks, have a low-fat diet yogurt or a couple of rye crispbreads with pure fruit spread or Marmite.

Alternatives   Keeping in mind these ideas, first, for fun, fill out our student's *Alternatives* column. Now, go back through *your* food diary and fill in your own *Alternatives*. What could you have done instead? You may not be able to think of alternatives for all the fattening things, but even if you can think of some it will make a big difference.

If, for instance, you have to travel around a lot in your car, on many occasions you could replace pub and café snacks with your own packed meal. You can buy insulated lunch bags so that everything, even yogurts, keeps fresh and cool. It's not beyond anyone who has basic facilities to prepare a healthy packed lunch or carry healthier snacks for nibbling when hungry. It is also possible to find alternative snack bars and cafés that offer less fattening, healthier alternatives. Ask around and take some time to seek these places out.

If you stay in hotels a lot, there are almost always low-fat things you can order. You are the guest and you can choose wisely from the menu. (For more tips on eating out, see restaurant section in Step Four.)

If you have to rely on another person – say, a parent or partner – to provide your meals, and those meals tend to be 'old-fashioned' high-fat-type meals, this may at first seem like an impossible problem to solve. Here, then, are my suggestions:

- Discuss with the person concerned whether it would be possible to have meals more in tune with the pyramid way of eating.
- Say that your doctor has asked you to lose weight and provide a weekly chart outlining the type of foods you need to eat (if it looks official, feelings aren't likely to be hurt).
- Ask yourself whether you could do more in the way of providing your own meals. By relying on someone else, are you perhaps being a bit lazy? If you offer to help more, might it not be a welcome relief for the main provider?
- See if you can do the food shopping, if not the cooking, and buy according to all the ideas in section 1.

- Ask for smaller portions of the 'old-style' foods and refuse desserts – eat fresh fruit instead.
- Eat low-fat, healthier breakfasts. Cereal, fruit, skimmed milk, yogurt and porridge are all good. By having a low-fat breakfast and refusing desserts, it will be easier to control your weight if you still have occasionally to eat an old-style main meal.

* * *

'I work shifts, which means organising a diet is impossible.'

Frequently I have listened to people who do shiftwork telling me that they can't lose weight because they have to eat an extra meal every twenty-four hours due to their shifts.

Step Four of the *Slim for Life* way of losing weight will show anyone on shifts how to plan a slimming campaign based on eating three, four, five or even six times a day. What matters is not how often you eat but what you eat.

I have also found that people on shiftwork (particularly nurses, who have one of the highest levels of overweight of any professional group in the country) nibble a lot on instant snacks such as chocolate, biscuits and crisps, 'to keep them going'. The solution, once again, is to plan ahead and take lower-fat nibbles to work (see suggestions in Step Four). Also, be content to lose weight slowly rather than not at all. You'll find more about this in Step Four.

* * *

'I'm on a low income, so I can't afford to diet.'

People who have spent a fortune in the past on fad diets and diet products always think that dieting is going to be expensive. Those who have lived on highly refined-carbohydrate diets – lots of white bread and butter, biscuits and cakes to 'fill up' –

and who don't buy fresh fruit and vegetables 'because they are expensive' have a very misguided idea of what you need to do to lose weight (this is in part the fault of sectors of the diet industry). If that sounds like you, you should read Step Three's section 4 (Say Goodbye to the Diet Mentality) carefully.

The fact is that a new-style pyramid diet is one of the lowest-cost ways to eat. It *can* be expensive if you want it to be, but look back at the pyramid on page 67. Bread, potatoes, rice, pasta, cereals: they are all low-cost foods. Pulses, too, are low-cost food. Fresh fruit and vegetables can be quite dear, but bought in season are not (especially if you're able to freeze them when there's a glut).

It's also the case that to lose weight you need to take in fewer calories than you did before, which means you should *save* money, especially on the high-fat, high-sugar, added-value lines such as chocolate, fancy cakes and pastries, sweets and ready-made desserts.

* * *

'I spend my life around food – shopping, preparing, cooking, clearing up.'

Perhaps you are a professional cook, or work in a cake shop; or perhaps, like millions of others, your family commitments mean that you seem to spend your life in the kitchen. I know so many people – mainly housewives and single parents – who never had a weight problem until they got married and began cooking for their partners glorious meals which they then felt obliged to eat too, or who have a tribe of children to cater for and end up eating most of the meals themselves.

If you have to cook for others, the best way to tackle this is to feed them as you would like to be fed yourself – that is, on pyra-mid-style food that won't make them fat.

You're in charge: if you're feeding them, it's up to you. Small children and teenagers have their own particular needs (for more on this, see Step Six) but, in broad terms, a reduced-fat, higher-carbohydrate diet will bring lifelong benefits to *everyone*.

So, if you spend much of your time cooking for people, think of it as a brilliant way to control what you all eat, rather than letting *it* get the better of *you*. Here are some simple tips that will help you in your effort:

- Try to prepare meals for others when you are not hungry.
- Batch-cook and freeze to save time and avoid temptation.
- Delegate wherever possible (e.g., ask someone to clear away leftovers that otherwise you might eat).
- Plan carefully and cook amounts suitable for the people you're catering for so that leftovers are less of a problem.
- Keep a bowl of low-fat nibbles in the kitchen for when cooking makes you feel hungry.

*   *   *

'I'm tied to the house all day and I get fed up – so I eat.'

'My marriage ended; I'm lonely and miserable.'

'I'm finding it hard to cope at work – and when I'm stressed or anxious, I eat.'

'Comfort eaters' use food as a friend. If you do this, remember that the circumstances which lead you to eating for comfort may not have been your fault, but that doesn't mean to say there is nothing you can do. You *can* do something – both about the eating and the situations that are causing it. It may well take time, you may win step by very small step, but you *can* take control.

Breaking the pattern of comfort eating
To deal effectively with a comfort-eating problem you need to do three things:

1. Realise that, long term, food used as a crutch is more of an enemy than a friend and recognise your comfort-eating sessions for what they really are. (For example, stop pretending you ate the food because you were hungry.) You must be honest about what you are doing.

2. Replace the comfort foods either with a less-fattening food that you would not normally eat for comfort, or else with a *non-food comforter*.

Food comforters Most people will find it easier at first to replace their comfort foods with less-fattening ones.

I have started off the list below with some typical comfort foods, alongside which I've also set out alternative less fattening, non-typical comfort foods. You continue this list by inserting your own favourite comfort foods and also, in the second column, some substitutes you like.

Chocolate wafer bar (200 calories)	Handful, ready-to-eat dried apricots (50 calories)
Individual fruit pie (220 calories)	Crumpet (80 calories)
Finger shortbread biscuit (100 calories)	Grissini stick (15 calories)
1 whole (full-size) chocolate Swiss roll (approx. 800 calories)	1 whole baguette, halved and spread with pure fruit spread (300 calories)

....

....

....

....

....

(For ideas on lower-calorie replacement foods, see pages 171–172 in Step Four.)

To make it easier to carry out this measure, it would obviously help if you made sure there are none of your old comfort foods at home and if you made certain you have one or two alternatives available. (See page 72 to refresh your memory regarding shopping tips.)

Non-food comforters These need to be things you can put into force immediately. They could include: **body treats** such as time to wash and blow-dry hair; smooth in body lotion; manicure and polish nails; deep-cleanse face; or redo make-up; **mind treats** such as reading a book you've been meaning to start for ages; listening to some upbeat music; exploring the stations on your radio that you don't usually bother with; or phoning someone you like.

If you feel particularly 'uptight' or anxious rather than, say, miserable or lonely or bored, the following are all good for relieving stress as well as replacing eating: a hot bath; soothing music; reading lightweight fiction; taking some exercise. This last is one of the greatest de-stressers of all, so either take a walk or do some deep-breathing followed by some floor exercises (for more ideas, see Step Five).

The great advantage of all these non-food comforters is that not only do they not make you feel guilty, as food comforters almost always do, but they actually make you feel positively better.

Note: Alcohol is not a good idea for long-term stress beating. If you habitually use alcohol – more than a glass or two a night – to 'wind down', you should consider seeking professional help.

3. Deal with the underlying problems that are making you so unhappy or worried that you need comforting. If these are problems that you can't, for now, find solutions to after reading to the end of this section and really trying to get to grips with, then continue to use the short-term replacement comforters as in point 2 and plan ahead for better times (e.g., *'I'm stuck in the house all day with two pre-school children and I can't alter* *that now, but when the youngest has started school I am going to ... ').*

ACTION

Keep a comfort-food diary, using your notebook, for at least a week, but longer if necessary.

Write these headings above six columns, leaving plenty of space for the last two: *Day, Time, Food eaten, Reason, Replacement strategy, Longer-term solution.* As soon as you have eaten something for comfort reasons, fill in the first four columns. When you have decided which alternative food or non-food comforter you will try next time you feel that same emotion, fill in the fifth column. Then try your best to think of a longer-term solution to that particular situation/problem/feeling that you can enter in column six.

Here are two examples of how you might fill in your diary:

Day: Wednesday.   *Time:* 7 p.m.

Food eaten: Whole packet of mini cookies.

Reason: Had tiff with girlfriend on phone when she accused me of something I hadn't done.

Replacement strategy: If this happens again, next time I will try to have a good cry instead; that often makes me feel better. Or I could hang up quickly and ring up my mum; she's always good with advice. Or I could phone my friend back straight away and try to explain how I feel.

Longer-term solution: I should think about my friendship with Pat. Why is she always picking fights with me? Can I help her behave differently towards me? Can I ask someone to find out why she is like this? Should I try to find a new circle of friends who make me feel better?

Day: Friday.   *Time:* 6 p.m.

Food eaten: Large bag of peanuts washed down by half a bottle of wine.

Reason: Had a really bad week at work; got home feeling I wanted to scream.

Replacement strategy: Cup of herbal tea and a sandwich would be almost as easy. Then I could read last week's fashion magazine while having a nice long bath. Or I could change into a tracksuit and go for a good walk in the park.

Longer-term solution: Should I ask for some temporary help in the office to ease the workload? Should I look around and see if there are other jobs that might suit me better? Or I could ask to be transferred to a different department. I don't mind hard work but the others don't seem to pull their weight.

If you are a habitual comfort eater you can't lose weight and keep it off successfully until you find ways to take control. And you *can* take control. You can say 'no' to the foods that are, ultimately, making you fatter and more miserable. But you should always try to work on the problems that are making you comfort eat all the while you are trying the 'alternative strategy' treatment.

If general loneliness and/or boredom is your main problem, here are some more prime suggestions on how to improve the quality of your life. If your self-esteem is low it may be hard to see how you are going to take up any of these ideas – in which case, turn to page 22 for help.

Long-term comforters   Could one help you?

- Give your time to people who need it – e.g., offer to get involved in local hospital visiting, or with the Samaritans, or fund raising in the community. Look through the Yellow Pages or your local newspaper for ideas on organisations to approach.
- If you're new to the area, visit neighbours to say 'hello'. Don't wait for them to make the first move. If you feel shy, use an excuse such as: 'Can you recommend a good electrician?' or 'Which is the best local greengrocer?'.

- Phone the local radio station and ask about people interested in forming a slimming club – perhaps based on the ideas you have discovered in this book – or any other kind of club run from people's homes.
- Join a penfriend club or write letters to people you know but haven't seen for ages.
- Enter competitions in magazines and see what you can win.
- Join a local hobby or special interest club – perhaps gardening or a choir, or the Lions if you are male. If you're stuck for ideas, think back to what you used to enjoy or, again, look through the Yellow Pages under 'Clubs and Associations'.

*   *   *

'With my monthly PMS, how can I control my eating?'

'My weight has rocketed since menopause.'

'I've got a slow metabolism.'

Eating the pyramid way – and following the advice in Step Four on planning your own programme around your circumstances – will not only ensure that you do slim but will actually help the PMS symptoms, which are certainly not all in your imagination. Hormone levels in women do vary tremendously according to the time in their menstrual cycle. Most women find it easier to eat less immediately after a period and up until ovulation; then there is a gradual increase in the need for food until the period begins. It is a simple matter to plan your slimming around this. Here are some more tips to help ease PMS and dieting problems:

- Consult your doctor to see if there is anything he or she can do for you and/or consider an alternative therapy (e.g., a herbal remedy)

- Eat 'little and often' during the days of PMS.
- Cut down on salt.
- Don't be too hard on yourself.
- Alleviate a craving for sweet foods with dried fruit, low-calorie diet yogurts or other favourites.

If you feel you generally have a 'slow metabolism' – i.e., you burn up calories less quickly than other people (and this may be why women put on weight in the menopause; their metabolic rate may be reduced) – dieting can seem to be a case of 'one step forward, two steps back'.

People's metabolic rates do vary quite considerably – for instance, a small woman aged sixty who is not very active may burn up no more than 1,400 calories a day if she isn't much overweight, whereas a 5 ft 9 ins (1.75 m) woman aged twenty with an active lifestyle or normal bodyweight may burn up 2,500 calories a day.

However, I should point out that:

1. Many people, particularly very overweight people, who think they have a slow metabolism don't in fact. All research shows that overweight people have higher metabolic rates than slim people (mainly because of all the extra work their system has to do in carrying around the extra weight and in 'servicing' the larger bulk).

2. People with a slower-than-average metabolic rate can do plenty to help speed it up (see Steps Four and Five).

3. Many people with naturally slow metabolic rates *do* manage to slim successfully and keep the weight off. All you need to do is tailor your slimming plan to your own needs (see Step Four).

REMEMBER!

If you have a busy or awkward lifestyle, don't give up! You can get slim and stay slim for life if you want to; there are ways round almost any problem, especially if you aim to lose weight slowly. It goes without saying that it would be much better for you to lose 2 lbs (1 kg) a month than nothing at all, even if you really want to lose 2 lbs (1 kg) a week. So do be realistic. You'll learn more about 'reasonable weight loss' in section 4 of this Step and in Step Four.

Lastly, try the following exercise.

ACTION

With the help of pages 171 and 305–317 (and by going round food stores if you are still stuck for ideas), write a list of your Top 20 Lifesaver Foods – snacks and nibbles that aren't high in calories or fat and which you can carry around and eat when you like. Set an upper limit of, say, 75 calories for each lifesaver.

Here are a few foods from my own personal lifesaver list:

ready-to-eat dried apricots (10 calories each);
diet fromage frais (approx. 50 calories a pot);
rye crispbread topped with Marmite (30 calories)
    or Tartex vegetable pâté (40 calories);
Grissini breadstick (15 calories each);
Crustini crispbread rolls (20 calories each);
fresh raw carrot slices with low-fat soft cheese for dipping
    (approx. 30 calories allowing 2 teaspoons cheese).

Don't forget that the items on your list, as well as being things you really like, do need to be both portable and fairly 'instant'.

Use your lifesavers on all those occasions when in past times you've succumbed to eating due to 'circumstances beyond your control'!

SECTION 3:

Be Your Own VIP

Other people, often especially those closest to you, can try quite hard to sabotage your best intentions to slim, as we saw in Step Two. This section will show you how to be your own VIP – the person *most* interested in yourself.

'People tell me I'm just fine as I am.'
'People say our family is meant to be fat.'
'People say I'm big-boned.'

Are you right to want to slim? If you have spent a lifetime – or, at least, a long time – listening to others tell you that you are fine as you are, it's time to decide whether or not they are telling the truth. To do that, you must make an objective assessment of your current weight.

The height/weight chart here is one I adapted from various others. I like to use it because its minimum weights are not too 'thin' (low) and its maximum weights are not too 'fat' (high).

Weigh yourself now, without clothes. Are you heavier than the maximum acceptable weight given for your height?

If you are much over, you certainly can do with losing some weight. If you are just within a few pounds, you could probably do with losing some weight, especially if your surplus is concentrated round your middle.

If your current weight is within the minimum and maximum range you may well not need to lose any weight, though as body shapes vary so much, even between two people of the same

HEIGHT/WEIGHT CHART FOR WOMEN

(Height without shoes; weight without clothes)

HEIGHT	MINIMUM ACCEPTABLE WEIGHT	MAXIMUM ACCEPTABLE WEIGHT
4 ft 10 ins (1.47 m)	7 st 1 lb (45 kg)	8 st 10 lbs (55 kg)
4 ft 11 ins (1.49 m)	7 st 3 lbs (46 kg)	8 st 12 lbs (56 kg)
5 ft 0 ins (1.52 m)	7 st 5 lbs (47 kg)	9 st 0 lbs (57 kg)
5 ft 1 in (1.54 m)	7 st 7 lbs (48 kg)	9 st 3 lbs (59 kg)
5 ft 2 ins (1.57 m)	7 st 10 lbs (49 kg)	9 st 6 lbs (60 kg)
5 ft 3 ins (1.60 m)	7 st 13 lbs (50 kg)	9 st 9 lbs (61 kg)
5 ft 4 ins (1.62 m)	8 st 2 lbs (52 kg)	9 st 12 lbs (63 kg)
5 ft 5 ins (1.65 m)	8 st 6 lbs (54 kg)	10 st 2 lbs (65 kg)
5 ft 6 ins (1.67 m)	8 st 10 lbs (55 kg)	10 st 6 lbs (66 kg)
5 ft 7 ins (1.70 m)	9 st 0 lbs (57 kg)	10 st 10 lbs (68 kg)
5 ft 8 ins (1.72 m)	9 st 4 lbs (59 kg)	11 st 2 lbs (71 kg)
5 ft 9 ins (1.75 m)	9 st 8 lbs (61 kg)	11st 6 lbs (73 kg)
5 ft 10 ins (1.77 m)	9 st 12 lbs (63 kg)	11st 10 lbs (75 kg)
5 ft 11 ins (1.80 m)	10 st 2 lbs (65 kg)	12 st 0 lbs (76 kg)
6 ft 0 ins (1.82 m)	10 st 6 lbs (66 kg)	12 st 4 lbs (78 kg)

height, without seeing you I can't be categorical. If you are, say,
a 5 ft 5 ins (1.65 m) female and you weigh 10 stone (63.5 kg),
that may well be a stone or more heavier than you *used* to weigh
even though your figures fall within the correct height-for-
weight limits.

However, what I can say with certainty is that if your current
weight is at or near the minimum weight given for your height,
don't consider losing any weight. You don't need to, though
perhaps you could do with some body toning – in which case,
read Step Five.

Now, if you *are* overweight, don't let people tell you that
you're fine as you are. It may well be that you are not fat enough

HEIGHT/WEIGHT CHART FOR MEN

(Height without shoes; weight without clothes)

HEIGHT	MINIMUM ACCEPTABLE WEIGHT	MAXIMUM ACCEPTABLE WEIGHT
5 ft 2 ins (1.57 m)	8 st 9 lbs (55 kg)	10 st 6 lbs (66 kg)
5 ft 3 ins (1.60 m)	8 st 12 lbs (56 kg)	10 st 9 lbs (68 kg)
5 ft 4 ins (1.62 m)	9 st 1 lb (58 kg)	10 st 12 lbs (68 kg)
5 ft 5 ins (1.65 m)	9 st 4 lbs (59 kg)	11 st 2 lbs (71 kg)
5 ft 6 ins (1.67 m)	9 st 8 lbs (61 kg)	11 st 5 lbs (72 kg)
5 ft 7 ins (1.70 m)	9 st 12 lbs (63 kg)	11 st 8 lbs (74 kg)
5 ft 8 ins (1.72 m)	10 st 2 lbs (65 kg)	12 st 0 lbs (76 kg)
5 ft 9 ins (1.75 m)	10 st 6 lbs (66 kg)	12 st 6 lbs (79 kg)
5 ft 10 ins (1.77 m)	10 st 10 lbs (68 kg)	12 st 10 lbs (81 kg)
5 ft 11 ins (1.80 m)	11 st 0 lbs (70 kg)	13 st 0 lbs (83 kg)
6 ft 0 ins (1.82 m)	11 st 4 lbs (72 kg)	13 st 6 lbs (85 kg)
6 ft 1 in (1.85 m)	11 st 8 lbs (74 kg)	13 st 11 lbs (88 kg)
6 ft 2 ins (1.87 m)	11 st 13 lbs (76 kg)	14 st 2 lbs (90 kg)
6 ft 3 ins (1.90 m)	12 st 4 lbs (78 kg)	14 st 7 lbs (92 kg)
6 ft 4 ins (1.93 m)	12 st 9 lbs (80 kg)	14 st 12 lbs (95 kg)

for your health to be affected ... yet. But weight tends to creep on gradually, so if you have, say, a 1-stone (6.35 kg) problem *now*, in ten years' time it could be a health-threatening 3- or 4-stone (19–25.4 kg) problem! By the way, the 'small bones/big bones' dispute is already taken care of: the wide difference in minimum and maximum weights allows for people's differing bone structures.

Okay, so, accepting that you *are* overweight, you might ask if some people are just 'meant to be fat'. If everyone in your family is fat, does that mean you should stay that way?

The simple answer is *no*. It could be that the whole family has a lower-than-average metabolic rate but, as we've already seen, that doesn't mean they have to be overweight. And taking an overview of all the available data on overweight in families, it is more likely that such a situation occurs because the family, as a group, eat too much of the more fattening type of foods and don't take as much exercise as other people. Research points to the probability that it is the eating *habits* that are passed on in families, rather than the predisposition to fatness.

*   *   *

'I have read that it is okay to be fat now, that people should be happy with the size they are. Apparently, it's not politically correct to want to diet.'

A lot of people, particularly women, are coming to me these days and saying they have acquaintances who tell them, or magazine articles and so on have pointed out, that they shouldn't be worrying about losing weight – that dieting is out of fashion and that being happy to be the way you are is now the trend.

Looked at from the health standpoint alone, that argument doesn't stand up, so I usually tell people who have been influenced by politically correct viewpoints that what they are being told is, in my opinion, very irresponsible and best ignored.

Believe me, keeping your extra poundage or stonage will do no good for any political cause. In the same way as getting slim if you can't add two and two won't help you to get a job as an accountant, staying fat won't enhance your chances either.

So if you are being made to feel that you are letting the side down by wanting to slim, have the facts about obesity and your health at your fingertips (see Step One).

Of course, it need hardly be said that if you are fat you shouldn't be treated like an idiot or a leper and it is important to stand up for your rights. This is one of the things this book is telling you: to assert yourself. Don't let anyone make you feel it isn't 'correct' to slim. Look at it logically: how on earth can it be incorrect to want a slim, fit, healthy body? We wash our cars, decorate our homes, groom our pets and cultivate our gardens. So what is so terrible about keeping our own bodies looking nice? If you think fat looks nice, that's fine, but staying fat if you don't think it looks nice isn't going to help you to be a better person.

Also, don't forget that virtually all of the people who say they are happy to be fat and so should you be are disillusioned dieters – people who tried for years to stick to a slimming plan and didn't. Many, rather than admit to what they see as a failure, say they have decided it is best to stay fat, and, of course, it makes them feel better about themselves if you stay fat too.

Focus your thoughts. As long as you aim for a sensible weight and slim in a sensible way, there is nothing wrong with wanting to lose weight. It's up to you: it's your body.

There is one part of the anti-diet band's argument I do agree with, however, and that is their claim that the media tends to overpromote the idea that women should be thin. Ironically, I don't think that the slimming magazines are the culprits here: it is the fashion editors (led by the designers and model agencies) who do this. Size 8 – the size of most of the new crop of fashion models – is not a size that most women could achieve, or would even want to. Thinness is not what you should aim for; you should aim for a reasonable size that you feel comfortable with and that you can sustain. Don't take any notice of fashion: women were meant to have curves.

Choose a reasonable target weight and, once you've done that, don't let any anti-diet argument dissuade you. The Department of Health is on your side; they have issued guidelines, in the 1992 White Paper on the health of the nation, for reducing the nation's obesity. This is because they know, as I know and you know now, that fatness can spoil life; fatness can cause illness; fatness can shorten life; fatness can kill. And the Government has at last realised that fatness costs the country a lot of money in lost working hours and in health care.

Anyone or anything that encourages us to sensibly achieve a reasonable body weight and to be fit is to be applauded, not condemned. To want to be slim is not to be neurotic or silly, it is to be rational and sensible.

*   *   *

'I'd like to lose weight but I never get any encouragement from the people you'd think would help me most – my family and friends.'

We saw in Step Two that at least some of the Very Interested People who will try to stop you slimming are your own friends and family; and we saw some of the reasons why. What can you do to alter their minds?

Here are some simple ways:

- Keep quiet about it. This advice is so obvious, yet most people don't even think of it. This time, don't bother telling anyone (except people who have to prepare meals for you) that you are going to lose some weight. It is something you have decided to do and there is no changing your mind, so why not just do it and keep quiet? By the time people realise you are losing/have lost weight, you will have proved to them that their fears were unfounded. You *haven't* turned into a diet bore; you *haven't* spoiled their fun; you *haven't* run off with a better-looking person than your partner and/or you *haven't* stolen your best friend's partner.

- Think of evolution, not revolution. Yes, of course, you will change in all kinds of ways if you lose much weight; otherwise there would not be so much motivation (see Step One). But if the changes in you are gradual, other people, and you too, will have time to get used to them. I've known ex-fatties who, on reaching their target weight, overnight change their hairstyle, hair colour, complete wardrobe and make-up, and then wonder why their partner gets jealous! It is better to make the changes one at a time as well as gradually.

● Stay cheerful. One of the main reasons why family and friends often hate the idea of their loved one slimming is that he or she is miserable. If you just carry on as normal in every way, there can be no cause for dissent or complaint.

Lastly, if you find it rather dispiriting that people you care about don't want you to lose weight, remember that they may have cause if you've complained loud and long on previous dieting attempts. And try to find people who *will* encourage you, or even join in with you. We all need support and help. Perhaps you could set up a slimming circle and get yourselves sponsored so that you raise money while you slim? Even if you're slimming on your own, you can find people to sponsor you. In fact, this is one way to make detractors change their minds: if they have an interest in how you get on, they will encourage, not discourage!

Five ways to say 'no' without saying you're slimming

● 'I've just eaten something, thank you.'
● 'My doctor says I've got to cut out fatty food.'
● 'I'm just not hungry at the moment, thank you.'
● 'It was delicious but I just can't manage any more.'
● 'I won't have a drink tonight, thanks – I'm driving.'

ACTION

Write in your notepad the names of people who you think are hindering your attempt to lose weight. Next write the reason you think they feel this way (this may take some thinking about – refer to Step Two, section 3). Lastly, write the solution (how you're going to deal with it). For example: *Name* My friend Sarah. *Reason* She was really strange last time I tried to diet. I think it may be because we're both about the same weight and she wants us to remain the same. Perhaps she'll feel insecure if I lose weight. *Solution* I won't say I'm slimming. When she notices, I'll say I'm just eating more healthy foods. I'll see if I can persuade her to change her eating habits a bit, too. If she loses some weight, then we'll still be the same!

If on previous occasions when you wanted to slim, the family caused trouble (sulks, sarcasm, etc.) – mainly because they were worried about their own menu – most of what has already been said applies. Just alter, in gradual stages, the way you prepare food and the types of food you offer; don't say you're slimming, and they probably won't notice, let alone mind. If, for example, one evening you decide to cook a new recipe from this book, you could casually say: 'I've tried a new recipe. I know you'll like it.' If you put the idea in dyed-in-the-wool, old-fashioned-style eaters' heads that you are offering a reduced-calorie, reduced-fat, healthier meal than what they are used to, they are bound to hate it, aren't they?

Five ways to keep the family happy while you slim

- Give hungry members of the family extra from the base of the pyramid – pasta, potatoes, rice, bread, cereals – and slightly bigger portions of the low-fat proteins, plus all the fruit and veg they can eat.
- Don't feel obliged to bake for them. One way round this is to give children a bakery allowance to spend themselves. Urge them to eat the doughnuts when you are not around! Another way is to make swops – e.g., wholemeal scones instead of Victoria sandwich cake.
- Cut down on the amount of biscuits you buy and also select a less calorific kind. When the barrel is empty everyone will have to eat bread or fruit.
- Avoid the martyr syndrome while you slim. Don't buy things for the family that you know you aren't going to eat – e.g., instead of a bought cheesecake (high-fat, high-calorie)

serve for dessert the new-style cheesecake on page 220, or a fresh-fruit fool.
● Be happy yourself.

* * *

'I keep reading that dieting is bad for you or dangerous. If this is true, it is a good excuse not to slim, but I do want to lose weight.'

You can rest assured that losing weight on a healthy diet and fitness programme such as *Slim for Life's* is not in any way dangerous. The risks are miniscule compared with the perils of staying overweight or getting fatter.

Losing weight only becomes risky when the method of dieting used isn't sensible. (Non-sensible methods are described in section 4 which follows.) I can assure you that, done sensibly, slimming:

● Doesn't leave you short of vital nutrients.
● Doesn't have an adverse effect on your heart or muscle tissue.
● Doesn't reduce your metabolic rate to a level lower than you would naturally have at your new body weight.
● Doesn't cause anorexia or bulimia (these tend to be linked to psychological problems and are highly unlikely to develop in genuinely overweight people who embark on a slimming campaign).
● Doesn't make you sluggish. Most people who lose weight sensibly report feeling sharper and more alert.

All these, and any other 'dieting is bad for you' hearsay, are the modern equivalent of old wives' tales. Disregard them.

SECTION 4:

Say Goodbye to the Diet Mentality

Has Dieting (with a capital D) been an important part of your life up until now? Have you conducted a love/hate relationship with your food and an ongoing battle with your willpower over a Diet campaign – a battle that, sadly, has so far ended in failure?

Here you can learn to leave that thinking behind you for good and begin to develop a more balanced and more realistic approach to getting and staying slim.

Although the rule for Step Three is 'take control', it is important to understand that 'overcontrol' is just as bad as 'no control'. Overcontrol leads to a fight with food and, almost inevitably, to long-term failure. So here's where you are going to learn to relax a little as you control not your diet but the wilder excesses of the hopes, expectations and resolutions that have been fuelled so long by the tyrannical diet industry. Here's where, once and for all, you rid yourself of the destructive diet mentality.

*   *   *

'I've already tried many diets – all fruit, liquids only, no food before noon, no protein with starch, etc. etc. and I've failed on all of them.'

Why do diets fail you? No, it isn't the case that you have failed on diets; the diets have failed you. They required you to be too tough on yourself and this prevented you from sticking to them.

Here are some of the reasons why these diets failed:

- You didn't like the foods they allowed.
- They didn't allow you the foods you like.
- You felt hungry too often.
- They didn't fit in with your lifestyle.
- They were ridiculous diets that, even if you followed them to the letter, wouldn't have worked anyway.
- They hadn't programmed you into a way of eating you could stick with – so any lost weight soon came back.
- After failing several times to help you lose weight, they made you feel you were programmed for failure.

The only way in which you 'failed' was in picking the diets in the first place, but, as you're not a nutritionist or health expert, how were you to know?

Also, have you succumbed to the power of the 'diet aid' ad? Have you tried mail-order slimming pills or any of the other 'cures' that promise weight loss without dieting such as slimming patches, sauna suits, special detoxifying potions, ear clips to stop hunger pangs, cassette tapes for slimming while you sleep, 'negative calorie' foods? Did you fail to lose weight on those as well?

'Diet aids' that promise weight loss without calorie reduction are not being honest and diets that don't fit in with you won't work. So stop blaming yourself and feeling inadequate. You can lose weight and you can keep it off just as well as anyone else can. All you need do is promise yourself that you will never try such a 'Diet' or 'diet aid' again.

Improving your outlook
To achieve the right frame of mind about slimming you need to recognise three things:

1. Weight loss does involve change – in the number of calories you eat; and/or the amount of exercise you take; and/or in the type of food you eat.

2. These changes need not be drastic and certainly need not be unpleasant.

3. For many people, changes in habits take time.

Don't think of losing weight as being on a diet. To slim successfully you must never, ever, wake up one morning (often a Monday morning, for some reason) and say: 'Oh help, day one of my diet!'

Yes, there are some people who decide they need to lose weight, embark on a diet, lose the weight and then get on with their lives. If you were one of those people, you wouldn't be reading this book. In your case there is *no* need to feel obliged to lose any set amount of weight during any particular timespan.

To overcome the diet mentality you need to:

- Start gently so you don't wake up one morning with that sinking feeling common to dieters of a tyrannical diet.
- Control your slimming campaign your way and don't take any notice of what other dieters you know are doing.
- Limit the fat content of your diet so that you can still eat plenty while you slim. Eating plenty is one of the keys to permanent weight control. The latest UK study as I write shows that people who diet on as much as 1,600 calories a day show better overall weight-loss results than people who try to keep to nearer 1,000 calories a day. This is because the people on 1,000 calories a day find it harder to stick to their diets (not because, as is often argued, low-calorie diets make you fat!).

  As long as your overall food intake is less – even if just a little less – than your energy output, you will lose weight. So in theory if you stay fat on, say, 2,250 calories a day, cutting down to 2,000 a day will still have you losing in the long run. Eventually you will have to cut down a little more, but that's another story (see Step Four).

- Set yourself a reasonable goal weight. If you have a lot to lose, this should be towards the higher end of the height/weight charts (see page 134–135) and it will also help if you divide the total amount of weight you need to lose into 'manageable bits' and 'mini-goals' (say, a stone (6.4 kg) or even half a stone (3.2 kg) at a time).

- Aim to reach your goal (or mini-goal) in no specific timespan. It isn't *necessary* to get there in any particular length of time; you just need to get there eventually. This way you will avoid setting yourself unreasonable weekly weight-loss targets. It is very easy to say: 'I will lose 3 lbs (1.4 kg) a week' and then, if one week you only lose 1 lb (½ kg), instead of feeling pleased at the 1 lb (½ kg) weight loss you feel you have failed. As this point the likelihood of you giving up is greater.

So if you do prefer to set a weight-loss target, it is better to choose a low one and to consider your weight loss over a period of a month rather than on a weekly basis. This is particularly useful for women who have menstrual cycles as weekly weight readings can give a very false picture both because of pre-menstrual fluid retention and because of many women's natural need to eat more in the week or so preceding the period.

* * *

'I'm either very good or very bad when I'm dieting. I can be strict with myself for days, but then the willpower evaporates and I binge.'

How can you beat the all-or-nothing syndrome? Alternating periods of bingeing and virtually starving are typical of an obsessive dieting behaviour pattern. Many women do this (the pattern differs from bulimia in that sufferers don't make themselves vomit). It usually isn't an 'eating disorder' as such, it is simply your body telling you that it needs more food. As I said in Step One, you don't *need* willpower if you're slimming correctly.

The low-carbohydrate, high-protein diets of the 1970s first caused the binge/starve effect to become apparent and many women have since been alternately crash-dieting and bingeing.

The fact is that if you starve your body of carbohydrate foods for any length of time, you will inevitably end up with a strong desire to eat the foods you've been avoiding. This is in part due to the fact that a low-complex-carbohydrate diet (low on foods such as bread and potatoes) can lead to a relatively rapid reduction in blood-sugar after a meal – a condition that makes us physically desire a carbohydrate food to restore the balance – and what will restore the balance most quickly is a 'simple carbohydrate', a sugary food such as chocolate, sweets or biscuits. This dose of sugar will send the blood levels soaring quickly.

Also, of course, it is well known that when people are deprived of something, psychologically they want it even more. Doctors have likened people on strict diets to tightly wound springs: the harder they try to stick to a diet, the tighter the spring is wound and the more pronounced the breakdown of the diet when that spring is released. So you see, this isn't you being 'good' or 'bad', it is simply you reacting in a normal way to an overly restrictive eating pattern.

Very low-calorie, low-carbohydrate diets are in fact the very worst thing you can go on for long-term weight control and one of the quickest ways to mess up your body's natural balance. Promise yourself you'll never again go on any diet that severely limits your intake of complex carbohydrates (bread, potatoes, pasta, cereals, rice and pulses) or that asks you to eat less than three times a day.

Here are the guidelines for avoiding the binge/starve trap in the future:

- Aim for slow weight loss.
- Eat plenty.
- Eat regularly.

- Don't think of any food as 'forbidden'; just remember to restrict some foods (the high-fat ones discussed in section 1) to sensible amounts.
- Always eat something nutritious when you feel hungry.
- Remember there are certain times when you may feel hungrier than usual. If it is real hunger (see page 108), don't feel guilty, eat.

PMS may make you feel hungrier than usual, and if your hungry patches regularly occur after your mid-cycle and disappear soon after menstruation begins, this is almost definitely the cause. Allow for it in your slimming campaign (for more help on that see Step Four).

*　　　*　　　*

'I find diets so boring that even if I start off with enthusiasm I tail off after a few days.'

'Dieting makes me depressed and miserable, so it's no wonder I don't stick at it.'

I am always amazed at the number of people who are convinced that to lose weight they need to eat certain types of 'boring diet food' – things like cottage cheese, lettuce, celery, grapefruit, bran and crispbreads – and to drink only lemon juice and mineral water.

Now, personally, I like all those things (except for the bran!) from time to time as a small part of my diet, but I can quite see that if that is your idea of a diet you will be bored. You may very well be miserable too.

Neither does losing weight have to entail living on the same one type of food – say a glass of milkshake – for weeks on end.

And yet the person with the 'Diet' mentality will hardly believe that you can actually lose weight without eating like

that. But that old idea that you must suffer misery and deprivation to attain a nice new figure is something to banish from your
mind straight away. It's not true and this book proves it.

Have a look through the meal suggestions and recipes in Step
Four. Do they look boring? Will you feel miserable and
deprived eating such a variety of tasty foods? Look at the
snacks list on page 171. You can eat all of those things too.

You will also find your local library and bookshop well
stocked with recipe books containing new-style, reduced-fat
recipes to try.

Give it a go! Forget the old image of a 'dieter'. You are a person who wishes to lose some weight and you are doing so. Losing weight is nothing more than weight *control* applied a little
more strongly. It isn't a secret land where only the fittest survive.
Neither are you locked into a routine you hate. You can lose
weight on the foods you enjoy best because, as we saw in section
2, there are plenty you enjoy that are also foods you can slim on.

Slimming isn't a prison or a desert island. It is you exercising
control in the way that suits you best. And knowing *why* you
have overeaten – as you have been discovering throughout
Steps Two and Three – is the key to knowing what does suit you
best.

*　　*　　*

'If I cheat even once on a diet and eat something that isn't allowed, that's it; I'm so disgusted with myself that I give up.'
'I never lose weight as quickly as I want to.'

When people talk about how they cheat on diets, it always
makes me think of school days and how strictness brings out the
desire to find a way to beat the system.

The point is that with the *Slim for Life* 'slimming campaign' rather than a 'Diet', you can't cheat because nothing is forbidden; therefore you can't feel ashamed of yourself and give up. So that's one problem solved easily.

There will, of course, be times when you will eat something you didn't really intend to eat. You can control these times by using the methods in section 2, but, being human, you won't eliminate them. What you must get out of is the habit of letting this panic you into abandoning your plans to lose weight. It's not logical and it's not necessary.

Remember that control is about being relaxed and happy with yourself – and admitting that you're not Superman or Superwoman! Don't expect miracles. Remember also that slim people sometimes eat high-fat, low-nutrient foods without getting fat and without feeling guilty. So, don't feel guilty.

Think like a slim person!

You are also in for disappointment if you have preconceived ideas about exactly how much weight you will lose, and exactly how quickly. For example, if you were 8½ stone (51.8 kg) in your late teens and you are now 9 stone (57.2 kg) after a successful slimming campaign but can't seem to get any lower, isn't that fine?

Don't expect too much. Always be realistic about what you can achieve and in what length of time. What other people can do is not your concern: we are thinking about what *you* can do.

Don't forget, either, that you can't expect to keep up the initial higher weight loss of the first week or two of your slimming campaign. That is because at first your body loses fluid called glycogen – a glucose complex in solution with water – as well as fat. When this glycogen loss disappears the reduced weight loss will be mostly fat plus a little lean body tissue. You will also, if you follow the advice in Step Five, be putting on a little muscle, which weighs heavier than fat and may therefore artificially reduce the loss that appears on the scales. So when judging your success it is often best to look in the mirror

STEP THREE ROUND-UP

There has been a lot to do and a lot to absorb in Step Three. But
I'm sure that you will feel by now that you *can* cope with losing
weight and face the problems you've met in the past with, if not
ease, much less difficulty than before. You may well have lost
some weight already by being more aware of your eating habits.
That's brilliant!

Now, if you can tick the following statements, you are ready
to move on to Step Four.

☐ I have recognised past 'failures' for what they really
were and they don't concern me now.

☐ If I learn new habits and practise them regularly, they
will eventually become old, familiar habits.

☐ I know that if I eat fewer calories than I 'put out' in
energy, I will lose weight.

☐ I am going to lose the weight I want to lose.

☐ I can do it, in my own time.

STEP FOUR

Eat to Slim

Losing weight your way

You may well have already lost some weight while you have been carrying out Step Three, but here in Step Four we will devise your own personal slimming campaign based on my unique 'Eat to Slim' plan. This plan allows you to fit your slimming around your lifestyle, letting you vary the amount you eat from day to day according to how you feel and what is happening in your life. As long as your 'eating to slim' days outnumber the other days, you'll still lose weight.

With the help of a large selection of pyramid-style meals and snacks plus tasty recipes, you'll find the no-hunger 'Eat to Slim' plan really easy to follow using all the techniques you've learnt in Step Three.

For anyone who has a set idea of what a diet is like (awful!) you will be amazed at just how pleasant eating to slim is!

YOUR BODY PROFILE

The first thing we need to do is work out your body profile so we can gauge your Optimum Eating Level. Answer the following, then add up your score.

Sex   *Score*

Male: score 3
Female: score 1
....

Age

Under 25: score 3
26–35:   score 2
36–45:   score 1
46+:   score 0
....

*Approximate amount of weight
you want to lose*

  5 st (31.8 kg) plus: score 4
3-5 st (19.1-31.8 kg):   score 3
2-3 st (12.7-19.1 kg) :   score 2
1-2 st (6.4-12.7 kg):   score 1
under 1 st (6.4 kg) :   score 0
....
(If you need help on this question,
turn back to pages 134–135)

Height

6 ft (1.82 m) plus: score 5
5 ft 9 ins – 6 ft (1.75-1.82 m):   score 4
5 ft 6 ins – 5 ft 9 ins (1.67-1.75 m): score 3
5 ft 3 ins – 5 ft 6 ins (1.60-1.67 m): score 2
under 5 ft 3 ins (1.60 m):   score 0
....

My total score is   _____

Now use your score to reckon your body type:

Score between 12 and 15: You are Type 1

Type one means that you are likely to have a very high metabolic rate and you should be able to eat more than the average person who wants to slim and still lose weight well.

Score between 8 and 11: You are Type 2

Type two means that you are likely to have a high metabolic rate and you should be able to eat a little more than the average person and still lose weight well.

Score between 4 and 7: You are Type 3

Type three means that you are likely to have an average metabolic rate. You will be able to eat well while you slim and lose weight at a reasonable speed.

Score between 1 and 3: You are Type 4

Type four means that you are likely to have a slower-than-average metabolic rate. The Eat to Slim plan will help you to lose weight but you should aim for a slow to steady weight loss and it is particularly important that you build more activity into your life (see Step Five).

My type is ....

Your body type is important because it determines both your likely weight-loss pattern and how much you will choose to eat on the Eat to Slim plan. As we saw in Step Three, if you are very overweight your metabolic rate is likely to be high, but your age, sex and height all have an important bearing, too. Put simply, the higher your metabolic rate, the more you should be eating on your slimming plan.

Many people who are very overweight find it hard to accept that they have a raised metabolic rate ('If I have a fast metabolic rate, why did I put on weight in the first place?'). But if those people were once slim (and all the other metabolism-boosting factors were average) their metabolic rate wouldn't have been particularly high. It is being heavy that causes the rate to rise. As you slim down, your metabolic rate adjusts and slows down too.

The reason the very overweight person should eat *more* on a diet is explained simply. Let's take an example. If you are, say, 4 stone (25.4 kg) overweight at 14 stone (88.9 kg), you have probably been eating up to 3,000 calories a day to maintain that body weight; by contrast, a slim person would maintain an average daily intake of about 2,000 calories. In scientific terms (and although bodies don't always behave exactly like this in practi-

cal terms, it is still a good guide), to lose 1 lb (0.5 kg) of body
fat you have to create a 3,500-calorie 'deficit'; so if you took no
extra exercise but simply ate 2,000 calories a day instead of
3,000, you would be creating a daily deficit of 1,000 calories or
a weekly deficit of 7,000 calories, which equals 2 lbs (1 kg) of
weight lost!

Therefore, a person weighing 14 stone (88.9 kg) at the start of
the slimming plan could lose weight at the rate of 2 lbs (1 kg) a
week while eating plenty. But if you were to do what many diets
tell you and start on 1,000 calories a day, yes, you'd create a
much bigger deficit and lose more weight, but by dropping your
calorie intake to only a third of what you have been eating you
would of course notice the big difference (even if you began
eating the pyramid way), and you would feel hungry and probably not stick to the plan.

As your weight reduces, though, you do need to consume
fewer calories a day as you approach your target. That is because,
as we have seen, your metabolic rate when you were very big was
artificially high, but as you get nearer normal body weight the
metabolic rate also reduces in accordance with your new size.
This means that in order to create that 'deficit' and continue to
lose weight, you need gradually to reduce your calorie intake.

By this time, you will have steadily become accustomed to an
intake of fewer calories and also to the adjustments in the type
of food you eat, so it won't be a problem.

Activity levels also have a bearing on your prospective
weight loss, so if you step up your energy output by becoming
more active you will lose weight more quickly (see Step Five
for all the reasons activity helps you to slim more quickly).

And one last point I need to mention about weight loss is that
in the first week or two of any slimming plan you can expect to
lose a lot more weight than in subsequent weeks. That is
because in the first week or two the weight loss consists partly
of fat but also of a lot of water, and glycogen (stored carbohydrate), which disappear as a natural reaction to reducing the

calorie intake. The glycogen balance stabilises after a week or two, but if you are very overweight it could mean that in the first week of even a reasonably high-calorie diet you lose half a stone (3.2 kg) or more. Even people with only a stone (6.4 kg) or so to lose will experience a 3-4 lb (1.36-1.82 kg) loss in the first week.

So don't think after a couple of weeks that because your weight loss is slowing down you are 'failing again'. You aren't. You are now losing almost nothing but fat, which is what you want to lose!

THE EAT TO SLIM TRIANGLE SYSTEM

We have established that the higher your estimated metabolic rate, the more you need to eat to slim, and with this in mind I have devised a simple system of meals and snacks, all coded with triangles, so that whichever body type you are – 1, 2, 3 or 4 – you can pick a plan to suit yourself.

Each triangle represents 50 calories, and for each body type there is a wide variation in the number of triangles you can have in any day, depending on what kind of day you want.

These are the four grades of day to choose from:

Optimum, Steady, Easy and **Relaxed**.

Optimum   An Optimum day is one that I consider will give you your best weight loss, being realistic. The number of triangles I suggest you eat on an Optimum day is the minimum amount I'd recommend you to eat on any day while you are slimming.

If you try to go any lower you won't be putting into practice all you learned in Step Three. *Never* slim with fewer triangles than your Optimum level!

If you choose the Optimum grade *every day* of your slimming campaign you will achieve the *maximum* weekly or monthly weight loss that I believe is suitable for you.

Steady   On a Steady day you will be eating more than on an Optimum day, but you will still be creating a good calorie deficit and will still lose weight – albeit more slowly – even if you decide to choose Steady days throughout your slimming campaign.

Easy   An Easy day is one on which you will be eating more than on a Steady day, but will still be creating a small calorie deficit and will still achieve a weight loss that can be measured in terms of pounds over a month, even if you choose Easy days throughout your slimming campaign.

Relaxed   On a Relaxed day you will be eating more than on any of the other types of day. You will probably be eating about the right amount to maintain your current body weight – i.e., you won't lose any weight if you choose a Relaxed day, but you won't gain any, either!

So all you need to do to continue losing weight on the Eat to Slim plan is choose more Optimum, Steady or Easy days than you do Relaxed days.

Here is the triangle guide for each body type:

Body type	OPTIMUM	STEADY	EASY	RELAXED
		Triangles per day		
1	30	35	40	50
2	25	30	35	45
3	22	27	32	40
4	20	25	30	35

Choosing your days
Remember, this is the slimming plan that YOU use to suit yourself. You suit your day's slimming grade to what is going on in your life and how you feel.

It is best to decide beforehand which grade you will adopt for the following day, but the system can also work beautifully to take away the guilt on days when you ate more than you intended – something that happens to everyone, no matter what size or weight. If you indulge too much, you can simply count that day as a Relaxed day and carry on with the plan. Remember that as long as you have fewer Relaxed days than other kinds of day over the course of a week or month, you will lose weight.

Obviously, the more Optimum days you have and the fewer Relaxed days you have, the quicker you will lose weight.

It's totally up to you how you combine the days. For example, you could choose nothing but Optimum days and Relaxed days. Or you could choose mostly Steady days and a few Easy days but no Optimum and no Relaxed. You could choose all Steady; or perhaps mostly Optimum but some Easy.

I suggest that you choose:

OPTIMUM days when you are feeling strong, positive and happy and the day is fairly ordinary; also, where women are concerned, in the early days of the menstrual cycle.

STEADY days for as much of the rest of the time as you can.

EASY days when, if you're a woman, you're heading towards the end of the monthly cycle; or when you know that, because of, say, business arrangements, it isn't going to be possible to do an Optimum or Steady day.

RELAXED days when you just want a day off or it's a special occasion.

I prefer to think of a slimming campaign in terms of how you do over the course of a month, rather than how you do each week – particularly for women because of the vagaries of the monthly cycle. But that also is up to you. If you prefer to divide your days up on a weekly basis, then do so.

Case histories

Here are some examples of how different people could use the Eat to Slim system to suit themselves.

- WOMAN, executive, with busy office-bound lifestyle during week but who enjoys cooking and socialising at weekends. Finds it relatively easy to eat to slim during the week so she has mostly Optimum days Monday to Friday, with an occasional Steady or Easy day. Saturday and Sunday she chooses mostly Relaxed days, with an occasional Steady or Easy day.

- MAN, company director, who finds the opposite works best for him. He entertains a lot for his company during the week but lives alone at weekends and finds it easy to prepare himself pyramid-style, eat-to-slim meals. He has two Relaxed and three Easy days during the week, then two Optimum days at the weekend. He isn't losing weight quickly, but he is losing weight!

- WOMAN, mother of two small children, and a part-time job on Tuesday, Wednesday and Friday when her children are cared for by a childminder. Finds it easier to slim on days when she is at home with the children so she has Optimum days Monday and Thursday. Can also do quite well when she is busy at work, so has Steady days Tuesday, Wednesday and Friday. Weekends she spends time with the family and enjoys going out every Saturday, so Saturday is usually Easy, Sunday Relaxed.

The system works well to help you over times when we naturally tend to eat more (e.g., Christmas, Easter, family holidays, anniversaries, etc). At Christmas, for example, you could give yourself several Relaxed days over the Christmas period itself, but in the busy run-up you would probably find it easy to follow a lot of Optimum or Steady days. Most people also find it easier to stick to Optimum days in summer and have more Steady days in winter.

On pages 164–167 you will find an Eat to Slim chart to fill in. This will help you monitor your first slimming month. When the chart is full, if you still want to lose more weight, copy it out into your notebook and carry on.

NOTE: Whenever you lose a stone (6.4 kg), you should go back and do the Body Type test again because, as your weight drops, your Type may change and you should adjust your triangles accordingly by rechecking the chart on page 156.

You could, if you have a lot of weight to lose, follow a broader plan than the monthly system. For example, you could lose a stone (6.4 kg) and then have a month 'off' with all Relaxed days; begin again to lose another stone, then have another month off, and so on. There is no law about how the weight should come off! Remember, you aren't 'on a diet' as such, therefore you don't have a 'diet' to come off.

'So how much weight will I lose?'

I don't want to give you specific 'weight loss per week or month' forecasts as, if you don't make them, that will invite again that feeling that somehow you have 'failed'. We are specifically trying to get you out of the 'tyrannical diet' mentality and into thinking like a slim person for life. Believe me, if you follow the Optimum, Steady, Easy, Relaxed system you *will* lose weight. And the more Optimum days and the fewer Relaxed days you have, the quicker you will lose. You should aim to have no more than fourteen Relaxed days in any month for successful weight loss. If the rest of the days in that month are Easy or Steady, you will lose a small to medium amount of weight; if the rest of the days are Optimum, you should lose a few pounds a month.

If you are Type 4 I do urge you to be content with a weight loss a month of a few pounds, and also to follow the 'weight loss per month' scheme rather than having a weekly weigh-in.

Look at it this way: if you have tried and failed to lose weight before but now you can lose, say, 2 lbs (1.9 kg) a month steadily, at the end of six months you will have lost a stone (6.4 kg) (some of which , in the first month, is due to glycogen loss) and nearly two stone (12.7 kg) over a year! A great success, I'm sure you'll agree.

Using the triangles each day

Now we have looked at the broad picture of how you will slim, let's examine the way you will use the triangles to give you a daily menu that you'll really enjoy. Again, there is plenty of scope for choosing the slimming plan that is just right for you.

All the meals, snacks and extras that follow in Step Four are triangle-rated. Supposing you are a Type 2 and following a Steady day, you have 30 triangles to eat. Below is an example of how you could use those triangles.

> *'I hate breakfast but I always want something mid-morning.*
> *I have to eat a packed lunch. My really hungry time of*
> *day is around 6 p.m., then I like a snack and a drink*
> *before I go to bed.'*

Breakfast: None, except some coffee and orange juice
   (1 triangle).
Mid-morning: A snack picked from the Snacks selection
   (4 triangles).
Lunch: A packed lunch from the Cold Meal selection
   (6 triangles).
Mid-afternoon: You should eat something at about teatime to
   stave off the hunger pangs, so have a snack from the Snacks
   selection (2 triangles).
6 p.m.: Have a hot main meal (8 triangles) followed by a fruit
   from the Fruit selection (1 triangle).
Supper: Have a bowl of cereal from the Breakfast selection
   (4 triangles).
Throughout the day: You use up some triangles in Extras –
   e.g., milk (4 triangles).

As you can see from all the triangle-rated meal suggestions in the pages that follow, you eat to suit yourself – big breakfast or small breakfast; large cold lunch or small hot lunch; main evening meal or light snack; several small snacks throughout the day and not one big meal at all .... The combination is up to you.

The only two *rules* that I'd like you to follow throughout your Eat to Slim campaign are:

- Always eat at least three times a day; preferably more.
- Aim to choose no more than 10 per cent of your daily triangles from the Red Extras list (see pages 183–189). That means, depending upon what Type you are and what grade of day you are on, you will be able to have from two to five triangles from this list.

Tips to help you

- Think about your 'hungry times of day' and plan your meals and snacks to fit in with them. Plan small snacks for times when you are least hungry.
- Don't be afraid if your body tells you it is hungry; if you feel the signs, then eat.
- If you plan to take exercise, don't eat a *big* meal immediately before, though a small-to-medium meal is allright.
- Begin the Eat to Slim plan gently. Start off with a few Relaxed days just getting into the swing of things. Then have a few Easy or Steady days before you begin on the Optimum days.
- The meal suggestions and recipes all follow, as nearly as possible, the 'new-style' pyramid philosophy, so you don't have to worry about that while you are eating to slim. The Red Extras give you your 'top of the pyramid' allowance of fat and simple sugars.
- Check through your store cupboard, fridge and freezer and run down your stocks 'old-fashioned-style' foods before beginning on the Eat to Slim plan.

- Buy only small amounts of the Red Extras so you can eat only small amounts!
- Try to plan ahead with your menus, using all the tips you've learnt in Step Three.
- Don't eat the Red Extras when you are hungry unless they form part of a bigger meal. Save them for after a meal.
- All the meal suggestions and recipes are based on my 'swops' principle, always using a lower-fat or lower-calorie food when it will do just as well as a higher one.
- If there is a food or snack you wish to include in your slimming campaign but it is not listed among the suggestions (see pages 168–191), then find out its calorie content (most commercial foods have a calorie value listed on the packet), count one triangle for every 50 calories and add it to the Red Extras list. If there is no calorie count given, look in at calorie guide, available in newsagents, or in the library. Or you could write to me, c/o my publishers, enclosing a SAE, and I will do my best to help you.
- I have tried as far as possible to provide meals that don't require much weighing of food, but you will need to weigh items from some of the meal selections – so check that you have a set of kitchen scales that mark $\frac{1}{4}$ oz (5 g) gradations. A set of measuring spoons is also a good idea, as is a measuring cup, since it's a much quicker method of gauging amounts.
- For those occasions when you eat out, there is a whole section of starters, main courses and desserts for you to choose from. Bear in mind, though, that the triangle guides are only approximate and that it is harder to stick to the pyramid method when you eat out. So class an 'eating out' day as a Relaxed day for the purposes of your slimming plan, even if you feel you didn't eat much!
- You may find it easier to stay with Optimum and Steady days if you plan plenty of meals and snacks based on the

'slow release' foods that take longest to be absorbed into your system. For instance, pasta, oats, most fruit, pulses, skimmed milk and yogurt are all 'slow release' foods, while other 'good for you' foods such as bread and potatoes are absorbed more quickly and may not keep you feeling so full up for so long.

- When choosing your daily menus, go for as much variety as possible so that you will get all the vitamins and minerals you need for good health.
- You can add Extras and Snacks to your main meals to make them bigger – e.g., add a soup snack to your lunch; or a fruit snack to your breakfast.
- Red Extras can be 'saved up' over a period of a few days. This is useful if you prefer one big 'treat' every few days rather than a little every day, or if you have a special occasion coming up and you know you'll want to feel free to eat or drink extra. If you want to save up your Red Extras in this way, keep a record in your notebook.

Long-term slimming

If you have a lot of weight to lose, you may find you want to widen the scope of your eating, perhaps by devising your own recipes, or by using foods mentioned on the following pages but in different combinations. In that case, please turn to page 221 at the end of the meals and recipes for the 'freestyle plan'. But you shouldn't move on to this until you have been on the basic Eat to Slim plan for at least two months and have recorded a successful weight loss.

Right! Now fill out the details at the top of the chart on pages 164–167, plan your first few days (remember, start gently with Easy or Relaxed days) and begin eating to slim.

EAT-TO-SLIM RECORD CHART – WEEKS ONE & TWO

My body type is: _____

My weight: at start _____ Day 8 _____ Day 15 _____

Day	Today's grade					
1		△△△△△	△△△△△	△△△△△	△△△△△	△△△△△
2		△△△△△	△△△△△	△△△△△	△△△△△	△△△△△
3		△△△△△	△△△△△	△△△△△	△△△△△	△△△△△
4		△△△△△	△△△△△	△△△△△	△△△△△	△△△△△
5		△△△△△	△△△△△	△△△△△	△△△△△	△△△△△
6		△△△△△	△△△△△	△△△△△	△△△△△	△△△△△
7		△△△△△	△△△△△	△△△△△	△△△△△	△△△△△
8		△△△△△	△△△△△	△△△△△	△△△△△	△△△△△
9		△△△△△	△△△△△	△△△△△	△△△△△	△△△△△
10		△△△△△	△△△△△	△△△△△	△△△△△	△△△△△
11		△△△△△	△△△△△	△△△△△	△△△△△	△△△△△
12		△△△△△	△△△△△	△△△△△	△△△△△	△△△△△
13		△△△△△	△△△△△	△△△△△	△△△△△	△△△△△
14		△△△△△	△△△△△	△△△△△	△△△△△	△△△△△

1. Record your body type, the corresponding number of triangles for each grade of day (see page 156) and your starting weight at the top of the page.
2. Decide which grade of day you will aim for each day and write its symbol (0, S, E or R) in the left-hand column.
3. Cross off or fill in each blank triangle as you use it. Use a red pen for 'Red Extra' triangles. (50 blank triangles are illustrated but your chosen day may allow less than that, in which case ignore the 'spares'.)

My triangles allowed are:

Optimum ☐ Steady ☐ Easy ☐ Relaxed ☐

*Fill in the triangles as you eat to keep
a check of your day's total*

Grade
achieved

△△△△△ △△△△△ △△△△△ △△△△△ △△△△△

△△△△△ △△△△△ △△△△△ △△△△△ △△△△△

△△△△△ △△△△△ △△△△△ △△△△△ △△△△△

△△△△△ △△△△△ △△△△△ △△△△△ △△△△△

△△△△△ △△△△△ △△△△△ △△△△△ △△△△△

△△△△△ △△△△△ △△△△△ △△△△△ △△△△△

△△△△△ △△△△△ △△△△△ △△△△△ △△△△△

△△△△△ △△△△△ △△△△△ △△△△△ △△△△△

△△△△△ △△△△△ △△△△△ △△△△△ △△△△△

△△△△△ △△△△△ △△△△△ △△△△△ △△△△△

△△△△△ △△△△△ △△△△△ △△△△△ △△△△△

△△△△△ △△△△△ △△△△△ △△△△△ △△△△△

△△△△△ △△△△△ △△△△△ △△△△△ △△△△△

△△△△△ △△△△△ △△△△△ △△△△△ △△△△△

4. At the end of the day, record which grade you achieved in the right-hand column (which may or may not be the same as you had intended).
5. Weigh yourself no more than once a week – for women I suggest less often may be better.
6. At the end of the four weeks, record your new weight, add up the numbers of each kind of grade of day you achieved and compare the total with your weight loss. Use the information to go easier – or perhaps try a bit harder – next month, or to stay on the same track.

EAT-TO-SLIM RECORD CHART – WEEKS THREE & FOUR

My body type is: _____

My weight: Day 15 _____   Day 22 _____   Day 29 _____

Day	Today's grade					
15		△△△△△	△△△△△	△△△△△	△△△△△	△△△△△
16		△△△△△	△△△△△	△△△△△	△△△△△	△△△△△
17		△△△△△	△△△△△	△△△△△	△△△△△	△△△△△
18		△△△△△	△△△△△	△△△△△	△△△△△	△△△△△
19		△△△△△	△△△△△	△△△△△	△△△△△	△△△△△
20		△△△△△	△△△△△	△△△△△	△△△△△	△△△△△
21		△△△△△	△△△△△	△△△△△	△△△△△	△△△△△
22		△△△△△	△△△△△	△△△△△	△△△△△	△△△△△
23		△△△△△	△△△△△	△△△△△	△△△△△	△△△△△
24		△△△△△	△△△△△	△△△△△	△△△△△	△△△△△
25		△△△△△	△△△△△	△△△△△	△△△△△	△△△△△
26		△△△△△	△△△△△	△△△△△	△△△△△	△△△△△
27		△△△△△	△△△△△	△△△△△	△△△△△	△△△△△
28		△△△△△	△△△△△	△△△△△	△△△△△	△△△△△

1. Record your body type, the corresponding number of triangles for each grade of day (see page 156) and your starting weight at the top of the page.
2. Decide which grade of day you will aim for each day and write its symbol (0, S, E or R) in the left-hand column.
3. Cross off or fill in each blank triangle as you use it. Use a red pen for 'Red Extra' triangles. (50 blank triangles are illustrated but your chosen day may allow less than that, in which case ignore the 'spares'.)

This month I achieved:

Total Optimum days _____   Total Steady days _____

Total Easy days _____   Total Relaxed days _____

Total weight loss for month _____

Fill in the triangles as you eat to keep   *Grade*
a check of your day's total   *achieved*

△△△△△ △△△△△ △△△△△ △△△△△ △△△△△ _____

△△△△△ △△△△△ △△△△△ △△△△△ △△△△△ _____

△△△△△ △△△△△ △△△△△ △△△△△ △△△△△ _____

△△△△△ △△△△△ △△△△△ △△△△△ △△△△△ _____

△△△△△ △△△△△ △△△△△ △△△△△ △△△△△ _____

△△△△△ △△△△△ △△△△△ △△△△△ △△△△△ _____

△△△△△ △△△△△ △△△△△ △△△△△ △△△△△ _____

△△△△△ △△△△△ △△△△△ △△△△△ △△△△△ _____

△△△△△ △△△△△ △△△△△ △△△△△ △△△△△ _____

△△△△△ △△△△△ △△△△△ △△△△△ △△△△△ _____

△△△△△ △△△△△ △△△△△ △△△△△ △△△△△ _____

△△△△△ △△△△△ △△△△△ △△△△△ △△△△△ _____

△△△△△ △△△△△ △△△△△ △△△△△ △△△△△ _____

△△△△△ △△△△△ △△△△△ △△△△△ △△△△△ _____

4. At the end of the day, record which grade you achieved in the right-hand column (which may or may not be the same as you had intended).
5. Weigh yourself no more than once a week – for women I suggest less often may be better.
6. At the end of the four weeks, record your new weight, add up the numbers of each kind of grade of day you achieved and compare the total with your weight loss. Use the information to go easier – or perhaps try a bit harder – next month, or to stay on the same track.

STEP FOUR ROUND-UP

When you are settled into your Eat to Slim plan (give it at least two weeks), you are ready to move on to Step Five and learn how to activate your body to help you feel great, look better, and give your slimming programme a boost.

See you at Step Five – but not until you're ready.

UNLIMITEDS

Use these foods and condiments in unlimited quantities while you are slimming and after.

Drinks   Black tea or black coffee (or with milk from Extras list); herbal tea; fruit tea (no added-sugar kind); water, mineral water; calorie-free 'diet' squashes and carbonated drinks (though try to keep these to a minimum).

Eats   Celery, endive, garlic, lettuce of all kinds, cress; pickled onions, yeast extract (Marmite etc.).

Condiments   Chilli peppers, chilli sauce (e.g., Tabasco); herbs, dried or fresh, all kinds; lemons and lemon juice, limes and lime juice; mushroom ketchup; mustard; oyster sauce; spices, dried or fresh, all kinds; soya sauce; vinegar, all kinds; Worcester sauce, tomato purée.

Note: Artificial sweeteners such as saccharin and aspartame may be used if you feel they will help you (but try to limit these to avoid artificially prolonging a sweet tooth).

CONDIMENTS

Within some of the meal suggestions that follow, 'condiment of choice' is mentioned. In that case, choose what you like from this list. (They are each worth half a triangle and are already included in the meal triangle ratings.)
All 2 teaspoons only unless stated otherwise.

Apple sauce; brown sauce; gravy (from stock cube), up to 3 tablespoons; gravy (thick traditional), up to 1¹/₂ tablespoons; mango or other chutney; horseradish sauce; oil-free French or vinaigrette dressing, up to 3 tablespoons; low-calorie salad cream; mint sauce; sweet pickle; sweet and sour sauce from jar; satay marinade from jar; Slim for Life Light Mayonnaise (see recipe page 192); Kraft Thousand-Island-Style Fat-Free Choice; Kraft Thick and Creamy Mayonnaise-Style Fat-Free Choice; packet stuffing.

VEGETABLES

Within some of the meal suggestions that follow, 'vegetable(s) of choice' is mentioned. In that case, choose from this list. (They are worth half a triangle and are already included in the meal triangle rating.) *Unless otherwise stated, the vegetables should be raw, boiled, steamed, braised, microwaved, baked or grilled.*

Alfalfa sprouts; asparagus; aubergine; baby sweetcorn; bamboo shoots; beansprouts; beetroot; broad beans; broccoli; Brussels sprouts; cabbage of all kinds and Chinese leaves; calabrese; carrots; cauliflower; celeriac; chicory; courgettes; cucumber; fennel; globe artichokes; Jerusalem artichokes; French beans and whole green beans of any kind; kale; kohlrabi; leeks; mangetout; marrow; mixed frozen vegetables; mooli; mushrooms; okra; onions (including spring onions); peas, fresh or frozen; peppers, any colour; radish; runner beans; salsify; shallots; spinach; spring greens; squash; swede; tomatoes; turnips.

FRUIT ▲

All the fruit portions listed here are each worth a maximum of one triangle. Cross a triangle off your daily chart (pages 164–167) only if you choose a fruit as a separate item. When 'fruit choice' is mentioned within a meal or snack, its triangle value has already been taken into account within that meal.

Apple, 1 medium; apple, stewed using artificial sweetener, max. 140 g (5 oz); apricots, fresh or dried, max. 5; blackberries or blackcurrants, stewed using artificial sweetener, max. 140 g (5 oz); cherries, fresh, up to max. 110 g (4 oz); clementine, 1; damsons, stewed using artificial sweetener, max. 140 g (5 oz); dates, fresh or dried, 4; figs, fresh or dried, 2; gooseberries, dessert, raw, max. 75 g (3 oz); gooseberries, stewed using artificial sweetener, max. 250 g (9 oz); grapefruit, pink or yellow, half an average; grapes, max. 100 g (3½ oz); greengages, up to max. 5; kiwifruit, 1; mandarins or satsumas, max. 2; melon, one good slice or half a small; nectarine, 1; orange, 1; peach, fresh or dried, 1; pear, 1; pineapple, 2 rings fresh or canned in juice; pomegranate, 1; plums, fresh, max. 2 or stewed using artificial sweetener, max. 140 g (5 oz); raspberries, up to 200 g (9 oz); rhubarb, stewed using artificial sweetener, max. 175 g (6 oz); strawberries, max. 200 g (9 oz).

EXTRAS

Add these to your menu as you want.

▲

140 ml (¼ pint) skimmed milk
2 rye crispbreads
2 tablespoons diet coleslaw
125 ml (4½ fl oz, one average glass) unsweetened fruit juice

▲▲

275 ml (½ pint) skimmed milk
200 ml (7 fl oz) semi-skimmed milk
1 slice bread from a large medium-cut loaf with a little low-fat spread
110 g (4 oz) potato, boiled, baked, or instant mashed
75 g (3 oz) [cooked weight] boiled rice or pasta equivalent to 25 g (1 oz) [dry weight]
(For Red Extras, see pages 183–189.)

SNACKS

Use these quick and easy snacks between meals or tack them on to a Cold or Hot Meal to make it bigger.

▲

- 1 slice French toast or rye crispbread with a very little low-fat spread and reduced-sugar jam or marmalade
- 2 Crustinis
- 1 Sunblest Crisproll with Marmite
- 1 Hovis wholemeal mini-loaf with 1 teaspoon reduced-sugar jam
- 1 fruit from fruit list
- 1 diet fruit yogurt
- 1 diet fromage frais
- 100 g (3½ oz) very low-fat set yogurt with 1 teaspoon honey
- 1 rice cake topped with 25 g (1 oz) low-fat soft cheese and tomato slices
- 1 tub Boots Shapers Fresh-Fruit Salad
- Selection of crudités plus 1 Grissini stick dipped in 1 tablespoon Kraft Fat-Free Choice Thousand-Island-style dressing
- 1 instant low-calorie soup plus 1 melba toast
- 1 can Weight Watchers minestrone soup

▲▲

- 150 g (5½ oz) natural low-fat or Bio yogurt plus 1 teaspoon honey
- Any two snack combinations from above list
- 1 Granose Apricot and Date Bar
- 1 crumpet with a little low-fat spread and reduced-sugar jam
- 1 small finger roll with a little low-fat spread and reduced-sugar jam or Marmite
- 25 g (1 oz) slice malt loaf with a little low-fat spread

- 1 large banana
- 1 mango
- 25 g (1 oz) sugar-free popcorn
- 1 Shape Twinpot yogurt
- 1 Weight Watchers soup plus 1 Crisproll

▲▲▲▲

- 1 average bap with a very little low-fat spread and 2 × 25 g (1 oz) slices extra-lean ham or with 2 low-fat cheese triangles
- 1 fruit teacake or bun with a little low-fat spread and reduced-sugar jam
- 1 large wholemeal pitta filled with chopped vegetables from list plus 1/2 × 113 g (4 oz) tub Shape Mexican-style cottage cheese
- 1 English muffin, toasted, plus reduced-sugar jam
- 1 pot ready-to-eat, low-fat rice pudding plus 1 medium banana
- 1 Boots Shapers Crispbread and Mushroom Pâté Lunch Pack plus 1 apple

BREAKFAST-TYPE MEALS

These vary from tiny breakfasts to big breakfasts. If you don't like to eat at breakfast time, perhaps you could have one at mid-morning instead (many are portable).

▲▲

- 1 diet fromage frais plus one fruit choice
- 1 diet yogurt plus 1 fruit choice
- 75 g (3 oz) natural low-fat yogurt with 25 g (1 oz) dried apricots or peaches or apples chopped in
- 1 Weetabix or 15 g (1/2 oz) puffed wheat with 100 ml (31/2 fl oz) skimmed milk
- 25 g (1 oz) bran flakes or Fruit 'n' Fibre (using milk from Extras list)

- 1 slice wholemeal bread from a large medium-cut loaf with a little low-fat spread and reduced-sugar jam or marmalade or Marmite
- 1 large banana

▲▲▲

- Unlimited ripe tomatoes, halved and grilled, on 1 slice wholemeal toast from a medium-cut large loaf with a very little low-fat spread
- 1 large banana and diet fromage frais or diet yogurt
- Unlimited mushrooms, grilled or poached in a little vegetable stock and served on 1 slice toast as before
- 75 g (3 oz or 3 good tablespoons) natural low-fat yogurt with 1 portion fruit from list, chopped, plus 15 g (1/2 oz or average handful) muesli or Bran Buds
- 25 g (1 oz or average bowlful) unsweetened breakfast cereal of choice – e.g., corn flakes, bran flakes, Fruit 'n' Fibre – with 150 ml (5 1/2 fl oz) skimmed milk or 100 ml (31/2 fl oz) semi-skimmed milk
- 1 small banana, mashed with a pinch of cinnamon and a dash of lemon juice, on 1 slice wholemeal toast from a large medium-cut loaf (no spread necessary), warmed under the grill for a minute
- 1 slice bread or toast with a little low-fat spread and reduced-sugar jam or marmalade plus 1 fruit choice or 1 diet yogurt or fromage frais
- 1 portion (125 g [41/2 oz]) fruit compôte, made by simmering dried mixed fruit in water to cover plus 2 tablespoons Bio yogurt and a sprinkling of bran flakes
- 140 g (5 oz) baked beans on 1 small slice wholemeal bread

▲▲▲▲▲▲

- 1 medium-cut, extra-trimmed back bacon rasher, grilled or dry-fried* until crisp; 1 × 75 g (3 oz) potato cake made by shaping instant mashed potato into a patty, dry-fried, *or* 75 g (3 oz) baked beans; 50 g (2 oz) mushrooms, dry-fried,

1 tomato, grilled *or* dry-fried; 1 wholemeal bap *or* 1½ slices bread from a large medium-cut loaf with a very little low-fat spread

- 25 g (1 oz) muesli *or* 1 Shredded Wheat with 125 ml (4½ fl oz) skimmed milk ; 1 slice wholemeal bread or toast from large medium-cut loaf with a little low-fat spread and reduced-sugar jam or marmalade; 1 portion from fruit choice *or* 140 ml (¼ pint) fruit juice
- 75 g (3 oz) smoked haddock fillet, poached or microwaved; 1½ slices bread from a large medium-cut loaf with a very little low-fat spread and 1 teaspoon reduced-sugar jam or marmalade; 1 portion fruit or 150 ml (¼ pint) fruit juice
- 75 g (3 oz) Greek yogurt topped with 1 teaspoon runny honey and 1 fruit choice, chopped; 1 average breakfast roll with a very little low-fat spread and reduced-sugar jam or marmalade
- ½ grapefruit; 2 low-fat pork (or pork and beef) chipolatas, grilled; 100 g (3½ oz) baked beans; 1 slice bread from large medium-cut loaf, plus a little low-fat spread

* *Dry-fried means fried in a non-stick frying pan which has been coated with a very little oil (preferably corn or sunflower, or you can buy a cooking-oil spray called Fry Light).*

COLD MEALS AND SNACKS

▲▲▲▲

- 75 g (3 oz) peeled prawns or tuna, chopped apple and 1 stick celery, chopped, all mixed with 1 level tablespoon mayonnaise dressing (see recipe for Light Mayonnaise on page 192, or use Kraft Fat-Free Choice), and green salad items of choice plus 1 medium slice bread
- Cheese and biscuits: 2 rye crispbreads, 1 cream cracker and 1 Crisproll with mixed salad of items from Vegetables list, plus *one* of the following: 25 g (1 oz) Brie, Edam, Port Salut or feta cheese; 2 reduced-fat cheese triangles; 25 g (1 oz)

reduced-fat cheese of Cheddar, Danish Blue or Cheshire type; 40 g (1½ oz) Dairylea Light; 50 g (2 oz) Shape low-fat soft cheese (⅓ of pack); plus a little low-fat spread

- 75 g (3 oz) [cooked weight] cold pasta shapes mixed with chopped apple or 25 g (1 oz) small seedless grapes plus 50 g (2 oz) chunks tuna in brine, drained, 25 g (1 oz) red pepper, chopped small, all tossed in oil-free French dressing
- 1 Boots Shapers Tuna and Pasta Salad
- 1 Boots Shapers Tandoori Chicken Sandwich
- Salad sandwich: 2 medium slices bread spread very lightly with Shape low-fat soft cheese and filled with as many salad items from the Vegetables list as you like
- 1 average soft bread roll filled with 2 thin slices (50 g [2 oz]) very lean ham plus 2 tablespoons reduced-calorie coleslaw (see recipe for Light Coleslaw on page 192 or use commercial brand) and sliced tomato
- Roll filled with 25 g (1 oz) reduced-fat Cheddar-style cheese plus lettuce, chopped spring onion and 1 teaspoon sweet pickle
- 1 Boots Shapers Turkey Salad Roll
- 1 Boots Shapers Soft Cheese and Hickory Smoked Ham Bagel
- 3 rye crispbreads spread with 25 g (1 oz) Tartex pâté (any kind) and topped with items from the Vegetables list – e.g., sliced cucumber and radish; 1 fruit portion from the Fruit list
- 1 half portion of Rice and Bean Salad (see recipe on page 196)

▲▲▲▲▲▲

- 1 whole pitta bread filled with 50 g (2 oz) hummus and chopped raw vegetable items from the Vegetables list plus side-salad garnish from Unlimiteds list
- Sandwich: 2 large (40 g, 1½ oz) slices bread with a little low-fat spread and filled with items from the Vegetables list

plus 50 g (2 oz) lean cooked chicken or roast pork or ham
and 1 item from the Condiments list

- Salad bap: 1 large bap with a little low-fat spread and filled
  with 25 g (1 oz) reduced-fat Cheddar- or Cheshire-style
  cheese or 1 hard-boiled egg, size 3, and plenty of salad
  items from the Vegetables list
- Sandwich: 2 slices bread from large medium-cut loaf filled
  with 1 × 100 g (3½ oz) can tuna in brine, drained and
  mashed, plus lettuce and cucumber; 1 fruit choice
- Bacon sandwich: 2 slices bread from a large medium-cut
  loaf filled with 2 tablespoons Light Coleslaw (see recipe on
  page 192) plus 1 slice back bacon, trimmed and well grilled
  then crumbled; salad garnish
- Ploughman's: 75 g (3 oz) slice French bread plus 40 g
  (1½ oz) reduced-fat Cheddar-style cheese or 1 whole 100 g
  (3½ oz) pot onion and Cheddar cottage cheese; 1 teaspoon
  pickle; tomato and celery
- 1 whole pitta bread filled with half a can of tuna in brine,
  drained, plus 50 g (2 oz) red kidney beans or other beans of
  your choice plus 2 teaspoons condiment of your choice (see
  list) and chopped salad
- 25 g (1 oz) Italian Mozzarella cheese, thinly sliced and
  arranged between 1 sliced tomato, topped with a drizzle of
  oil-free French dressing and garnished with sliced black
  olives and spring onions; plus 75 g (3 oz) slice French bread
- Takeaway: 1 Boots Shapers Back Bacon and Cream Cheese
  Bloomer, plus 1 apple; or 1 Boots Shapers Brie and Black
  Grape Sandwich, plus a fruit choice; or any chicken salad
  (no mayonnaise) or ham-and-tomato sandwich; or pastrami
  and tomato bagel; or Marks and Spencer Tandoori Chicken
  or Chicken Tikka pitta
- Salade Niçoise (see recipe on page 193) plus 1 slice bread
  from a medium-cut large loaf
- Hawaiian Rice Salad with Chicken or with vegetarian option
(see recipe on page 194)

▲▲▲▲▲▲▲▲

- Triple-decker sandwich: 3 slices bread from a large medium-cut loaf lightly spread with low-fat spread and the first layer filled with 40 g (1½ oz) extra-lean ham and the second layer with 40 g (1½ oz) cooked chicken or 1 medium hard-boiled egg, both layers with lettuce, cress and tomato plus 1 condiment of your choice
- Ploughman's: 75 g (3 oz) French bread with a little low-fat spread; 40 g (1½ oz) reduced-fat Cheddar or Cheshire-style cheese or Brie; 2 teaspoons sweet pickle; 2 pickled onions; a large mixed salad of items from the Vegetables and Unlimiteds lists
- Sandwich: 2 large slices bread with a little low-fat spread, filled with 50 g (2 oz) cooked chicken mixed with 1 tablespoon Light Mayonnaise (see recipe on page 192) plus plenty of vegetable items; 1 fruit choice; 1 medium banana
- Salad platter: 200 g (7 oz) cold cooked new potatoes tossed in 1 tablespoon Light Mayonnaise (see recipe on page 192), *or* 125 g (4½ oz) cooked rice and chopped peppers tossed in oil-free French dressing; 50 g (2 oz, 2 average slices) lean roast beef or pork or very lean cooked ham; mixed salad of items from Vegetables list; condiment of your choice
- Pasta Salad with Crispy Bacon (see recipe on page 194)
- Rice and Bean Salad (see recipe on page 196)

▲▲▲▲▲▲▲▲▲▲

- Ploughman's: 100 g (3½ oz) piece French bread with a little low-fat spread; 50 g (2 oz) Brie or reduced-fat Cheddar *or* 25 g (1 oz) regular Cheddar or Stilton; 2 teaspoons sweet pickle; tomato, celery, onion rings and lettuce
- Salad platter: 225 g (8 oz) cold cooked new potatoes tossed in 1 tablespoon Light Mayonnaise (see recipe on page 192) or Kraft Mayonnaise-style Fat-Free Choice; salad of 50 g (2 oz) cold cooked sweetcorn mixed with 1 small chopped

red pepper and oil-free French dressing; salad greens; 75 g
(3 oz) very lean cold roast beef or pork or lean cooked ham
or 100 g (3½ oz) cold cooked chicken (no skin) or turkey;
plus 1 condiment of your choice (see list)

- 100 g (3½ oz) cold cooked chicken (no skin) chopped and
  mixed with 1½ tablespoons Light Mayonnaise (see recipe
  on page 192) or Kraft Mayonnaise-style Fat-Free Choice
  which has been blended with 1 teaspoon mild curry powder
  and 1 teaspoon mango chutney; green salad; 75 g (3 oz)
  French bread
- Prawn and Pasta Salad (see recipe on page 195)
- Rice and Bean Salad (see recipe on page 196) with 1
  chopped hard-boiled egg added

HOT MEALS AND SNACKS

▲▲▲▲

- Any Weight Watchers canned soup plus 1 slice bread from a
  large medium-cut loaf; 1 fruit portion of choice
- 1 slice bread from a large medium-cut loaf toasted and
  spread with a little low-fat spread and topped with 1
  medium poached egg *or* 140 g (5 oz, third of a can) baked
  beans *or* wholewheat spaghetti in tomato sauce
- 1 × 50 g (2 oz) beefburger, well grilled, in 1 average bap
  plus salad items from the Vegetables list and lettuce; 1
  condiment of your choice (see list)
- 1 × 175 g (6 oz) baked potato split and topped with 1 good
  tablespoon 8% fat natural fromage frais and chopped chives
- 1 portion of Ratatouille (see recipe on page 197) with 1
  average roll
- 1 slice bread from a large medium-cut loaf toasted and
  topped with 40 g (1½ oz) grated reduced-fat Cheddar-style
  cheese and sliced tomato and grilled until bubbling
- 1 can Campbell's Vegetable and Pasta Main Course soup;
  fruit portion of your choice

- 1 portion of Tangy Tomato Soup (see recipe on page 198) with 1 small roll
- Mulligatawny with beans: heat one 300 g (10½ oz) can Heinz oxtail soup with 1 level teaspoon mild curry powder and 50 g (2 oz) cooked beans of your choice (e.g., pinto, black-eye) or cooked brown lentils

▲▲▲▲▲▲

- 550 ml (1 pint) lentil and vegetable or lentil and tomato soup (e.g., New Covent Garden) plus 1 large (40 g [1½ oz]) slice bread
- 1 × 225 g (8 oz) baked potato filled with 140 g (5 oz) baked beans or chilli beans
- 1 × 225 g (8 oz) can Heinz barbecue beans on 1 large (40 g [1½ oz]) slice toast
- 175 g (6 oz) new or boiled or mashed potatoes; a large serving of any choice from the Vegetables list; 150 g (5½ oz) white fish of your choice simmered in a non-stick pan with a little white wine or a dash of wine vinegar mixed with 1 tablespoon water plus 1 firm tomato, chopped and 2 spring onions, chopped. Simmer until fish is tender
- Selection of vegetables of your choice from the list, cut into strips and stir-fried in a non-stick pan in 2 teaspoons oil, 1 condiment and spices of your choice, with 1 medium egg added and stir-fried at last minute. Serve on 40 g (1½ oz) [dry weight] egg thread noodles, soaked according to instructions, or on the same weight of boiled rice
- 175 g (6 oz) mashed or baked potato with 1 medium serving of peas or sweetcorn or baked beans plus 1 portion of cod steak in parsley sauce or 150 g (5½ oz) any white fish baked in foil with herbs and lemon juice
- 1 × 100 g (4 oz) portion of New-Style Roast Potatoes (see recipe on page 198) with 2 portions of vegetables from the list and 1 small breast of chicken (no skin), baked
- Chicken Salsa Tacos (see recipe on page 199)

- Rice-Stuffed Baked Vegetables (see recipe on page 200)
- Italian-Style Roast Vegetables with accompaniment (see recipe on page 201)
- Indonesian Stir-Fry (see recipe on page 202)
- Chinese Beef and Red Pepper Stir-Fry (see recipe on page 203)
- 50 g (2 oz) [dry weight] pasta of your choice boiled and topped with 1 portion of Tomato Sauce (see recipe on page 204) plus 1 level tablespoon Parmesan cheese

▲▲▲▲▲▲▲▲▲

- 1 portion of Ratatouille (see recipe on page 197) mixed with 65 g (2½ oz) [dry weight] pasta of your choice boiled and topped with 1 tablespoon grated Parmesan or 2 tablespoons Mozzarella cheese
- 1 × 100 g (3½ oz) gammon or bacon steak grilled and topped with 1 slice pineapple plus 75 g (3 oz) sweetcorn or peas, 175 g (6 oz) new potatoes and 1 condiment of your choice; 1 fruit choice
- 1 average beefburger, well grilled, in 1 burger bun plus 1 condiment of your choice; 75 g (3 oz) oven chips; a large mixed salad of items from the Vegetables list plus Unlimiteds
- 1 × 175 g (6 oz) baked potato *or* 100 g (3½ oz) New-Style Roast Potatoes (see recipe on page 198); 1 medium chicken portion (no skin), baked (try using fresh rosemary and thyme with lemon juice to flavour); 1 portion of peas or sweetcorn; up to 2 portions of vegetables of your choice from the list; 1 condiment of your choice; 1 fruit choice
- Peppered lamb: 1 × 100 g (3½ oz) lamb steak with crushed peppercorns pressed into surface both sides, grilled; 225 g (8 oz) baked potato; either a large mixed salad or 2 portions of vegetables of your choice from the list
- 1 average pink trout fillet cooked in a non-stick pan in 1 teaspoon low-fat spread with 1 tablespoon chopped

almonds added at last minute; 2 portions of vegetables of
your choice from the list; 125 g (4½ oz) new or boiled
potatoes

- 2 ready-made savoury pancakes (crêpes) filled with 1 portion
  of Chicken Salsa mixture (see recipe on page 199); a large
  mixed salad of items from the Vegetables and Unlimited lists
- Vegetable omelette: beat two medium eggs with seasoning
  and cook in a non-stick pan that you've coated with a
  brushing of oil, adding a variety of lightly cooked and
  chopped vegetables of your choice (e.g., courgettes, onion,
  leek) or raw salad vegetables (e.g., peppers, tomato, spring
  onion). Turn carefully halfway through cooking and serve
  flat with 1 large wholemeal roll or 50 g (2 oz) slice French
  bread and side salad
- Bean and bacon hotpot: grill well 1 lean slice back bacon
  and crumble it into a saucepan with 1 × 225 g (8 oz) can
  barbecued baked beans; heat and serve with 1 large
  wholemeal roll or 2 slices bread from a medium loaf
- Cauliflower and Bacon Gratin (see recipe on page 205)
  served with 40 g (1½ oz) hunk of bread
- Jambalaya (see recipe on page 206)
- Seafood Tagliatelle (see recipe on page 207)
- Spiced Pork with Rice (see recipe on page 208)
- Sweet and Sour Stir-Fry (see recipe on page 209)
- Seafood Crumble (see recipe on page 210) with 175 g (6 oz)
  new or instant mashed potatoes and green salad or green
  beans

▲▲▲▲▲▲▲▲▲▲

- 1 small ready-made pizza base topped with 1 portion of
  Tomato Sauce (see recipe on page 204) or half a ready-
  made jar of sauce, covered with 2 tablespoons grated
  Mozzarella cheese and a selection of sliced vegetables of
  your choice – e.g., mushroom, tomato, pepper, onion; serve
  with salad

- 4 ready-prepared barbecued spare ribs, baked or grilled and served with 50 g (2 oz) [dry weight] rice, boiled, plus 1 condiment of your choice and plenty of salad
- 1 × 225 g (8 oz) baked potato with 75 g (3 oz) lean roast beef or lamb or grilled steak or liver *or* 110 g (4 oz) lean roast pork or chicken; 2 portions of vegetables from the list; 1 condiment of your choice
- Beef and Vegetable Curry with Rice (see recipe on page 211)
- Vegetable Lasagne (see recipe on page 212)
- Pasta Spirals with Minced Beef and Vegetables (see recipe on page 213)
- Chilli Con Carne and Rice (see recipe on page 214)
- Chicken and Mushroom Risotto (see recipe on page 215)
- Pasta and Tuna Bake (see recipe on page 217)
- 3 low-fat pork chipolatas, grilled and served with 150 g (5½ oz) baked beans and 175 g (6 oz) instant mashed potato plus 1 condiment of your choice

▲▲▲▲▲▲▲▲▲▲▲▲

- Luxury Paella (see recipe on page 216)
- Double portion of any of the 6–▲ meals

DESSERTS

▲

- 1 portion of fresh fruit from the list
- 1 individual diet fruit fromage frais (e.g., Boots Shapers)
- 1 individual diet fruit yogurt (e.g., Shape)
- 100 g (3½ oz) low-fat natural yogurt

▲▲

- 1 portion (up to 225 g, 8 oz) of fresh fruit salad with a squirt of aerosol cream
- 1 banana (cold or baked in foil with a little orange juice) plus a squirt of aerosol cream

- 50 ml (2 fl oz) ice-cream substitute (e.g., 'Too Good to be True') with 1 portion of fresh fruit from the list
- 1 Shape Twinpot
- Strawberry fool made by whipping 110 g (4 oz) fresh strawberries, hulled and chopped, with 100 g (3½ oz) natural fromage frais and a level teaspoon of fructose
- 1 Boots Shapers Raspberry Trifle
- 1 Boots Shapers Peach Sundae

▲▲▲

- 25 g (1 oz) dried apricots or peaches simmered in 50 ml (2 fl oz) water for 30 minutes then mashed including juices and served in the base of a wineglass topped with 2 tablespoons Greek yogurt and sprinkled with 1 tablespoon grapenuts
- 1 portion of Blackcurrant Cheesecake (see recipe on page 220)

▲▲▲▲

- 1 portion of Fruit-Filled Flan (see recipe on page 218)
- 1 Fruit Pancake with Creamy Sauce (see recipe on page 219)

RED EXTRAS

Biscuits

▲

1 fig-roll biscuit
1 Jaffa cake
1 chocolate chip cookie
2 Nice biscuits
1 gingernut biscuit
1 Bourbon biscuit

▲▲

1 Breakaway Milk biscuit
1 shortbread finger

1 Yo Yo biscuit
3 Rich Tea biscuits
3 cream crackers
1 Harvest Chewy or Crunchy bar

▲▲▲

1 Jordan's cereal bar
1 Penguin biscuit
1 Granose carob-coated fruit bar
1 Boots chocolate-coated cereal bar
2 Hobnob biscuits
2 digestive biscuits
1 Hobnob bar
2 chocolate digestive biscuits

▲▲▲▲

1 Chocolate Chip Tracker
1 Roast Nut Tracker

Chocolates and Sweets

▲

1 chocolate from assortment
1 toffee from assortment

▲▲

1 Lo Bar
1 fun-size Double-Decker
2 fingers Kit Kat
1 × 20 g (³⁄₄ oz) Cadbury's Dairy Milk bar
1 fun-size pack Maltesers
1 small bar soft nougat
1 tube Polo mints

▲▲▲

1 Cadbury's Fudge
2-bar Twix Teabreak
2 fun-size Wispas

35 g (1¼ oz) bag Revels
1 tube fruit gums or pastilles

▲▲▲▲

1 standard Crunchie
1 Wispa
1 Cadbury's Cream Egg
1 Cadbury's Flake
1 tube Toffos
1 tube Smarties
1 Aero Chunky
1 standard (40 g, 1½ oz) bag Maltesers

▲▲▲▲▲

1 Cadbury's Caramel
1 standard Cadbury's Dairy Milk bar
1 standard Cadbury's bar Fruit and Nut
1 Lion bar
1 Picnic
1 tube Rolos

Desserts, Gâteaux, Ices

▲▲

- 1 × 125 g (4½ oz) French-style set yogurt
- 1 ice lolly
- 1 soft ice cream in cone
- 1 meringue nest filled with fresh fruit and a squirt of aerosol cream
- 1 × 150 g (5½ oz) pot Ambrosia low-fat custard or rice pudding
- 1 Bailey's Puddi
- 1 individual strawberry mousse
- 1 Boots Shapers fruit fool
- 1 × 100 ml (3½ oz) low-calorie ice cream or ice cream substitute plus 1 flat wafer

▲▲▲

- 1 Cadbury's Dairy Milk mousse
- 1 individual pot crème caramel
- 1 individual trifle
- 1 St Ivel Black Forest dessert
- 1 portion of Blackcurrant Cheesecake (see recipe on page 220)
- 1 × 150 g (5½ oz) tub Bio or fruit yogurt or Greek yogurt
- 1 × 100 g (3½ oz) tub fruit fromage frais

▲▲▲▲

- 1 × 100 g (3½ oz) slice Sara Lee Lite Cheesecake
- 1 × 100 g (3½ oz) slice single-crust apple pie with 2 tablespoons low-fat custard or Shape single cream
- 1 King Cone or Cornetto
- 1 Mars or Snickers ice cream
- 1 Thick and Creamy yogurt or Duet (twinpot) yogurt

▲▲▲▲▲

- 1 individual St Ivel cheesecake
- 1 × 75 g (3 oz) slice Black Forest gâteau or similar

Cakes and Bakery

▲▲

- 1 Mr Kipling French or Fruit Fancy

▲▲▲

- Bird's Eye Dairy Cream Eclair (frozen)
- 1 jam tart
- 1 small croissant
- 1 average slice carrot (passion) cake

▲▲▲▲

- 1 iced finger bun
- 1 average slice jam sponge
- 1 individual apple pie
- 1 average slice rich fruit cake

▲▲▲▲▲
- 1 jam doughnut
- 1 average slice chocolate cake

Alcohol and Drinks

▲

- 1 glass low-alcohol wine
- 1 average measure sherry
- 1 single measure spirits

▲▲

- 1 medium glass dry or medium wine
- 1 small glass sweet wine
- 275 ml (½ pint) beer or lager
- 275 ml (½ pint) cider
- 1 liqueur
- 1 can lemonade

▲▲▲

- 1 can coke

Sugar and Spreads

▲

- 2 heaped or 3 level teaspoons sugar
- 3 teaspoons honey or syrup or jam
- 2 teaspoons chocolate spread or peanut butter

Savouries

▲

- 1 heaped tablespoon grated Parmesan cheese
- 2 heaped tablespoons grated reduced-fat Cheddar or Mozzarella

▲▲

- 25 g (1 oz) full-fat cream cheese or Cheddar cheese or Stilton or Blue Brie
- 40 g (1½ oz) Edam or Brie or reduced-fat Cheddar

▲▲▲

- 1 packet crisps (25 or 28 g, 1 oz size)

▲▲▲▲

- 100 g (3½ oz) small portion average-cut chips

▲▲▲▲▲

- 1 samosa
- 1 spring roll

▲▲▲▲▲▲

- 1 standard-size Scotch egg
- 1 standard-size sausage roll
- 1 × 110 g (4 oz) slice quiche
- 1 buffet (party-size) pork pie

▲▲▲▲▲▲▲▲

- 1 average (150 g, 5½ oz) Cornish pasty

Fats and High-fat Items

▲

- 1 good tablespoon double cream
- 1 tablespoon reduced-calorie mayonnaise
- 15 g (½ oz) low-fat spread

▲▲

- 1 tablespoon full-fat mayonnaise
- 1 tablespoon French dressing
- 100 ml (3½ fl oz, average serving) custard
- 25 g (1 oz) low-fat spread
- 140 ml (¼ pint) full cream milk

▲▲▲

- 1 tablespoon oil, any kind
- 25 g (1 oz) creamed coconut
- 25 g (1 oz) taramasalata

▲▲▲▲

- 25 g (1 oz) butter
- 25 g (1 oz) margarine – any kind, including polyunsaturated, unless labelled 'low fat'

EATING OUT AND TAKEAWAYS

Starters

▲

- Fruit juice
- Plain melon
- Grapefruit
- Consommé

▲▲

- Vegetable soup – any kind except 'cream of'
- Marinated mushrooms
- Chinese-style soup (e.g., crab and sweetcorn)

▲▲▲▲

- French onion soup or minestrone
- Asparagus with butter
- Onion bhaji
- Samosa, small
- Stuffed mushrooms or tomatoes

▲▲▲▲▲▲

- Prawn cocktail (bread not included)
- Pâté and toast
- Avocado with prawns or vinaigrette
- 2 Chinese spare ribs
- Average Greek meze platter
- Taramasalata and pitta

Main Courses

▲▲▲▲▲▲

- Regular hamburger in bun from takeaway (no chips)
- Half a 10-inch (25 cm) pizza
- Grilled fish; new potatoes; green vegetables
- Grilled breast of chicken; new potatoes; salad

▲▲▲▲▲▲▲▲

- Individual pizza (5-inch, 12 cm deep or 7-inch, 18 cm crispy)
- McChicken sandwich
- Quarterpounder hamburger with bun
- Dolmades (stuffed vine leaves)
- Kebab and salad
- Mixed vegetable or prawn chop suey

▲▲▲▲▲▲▲▲▲▲

- 200 g (7 oz) steak or gammon steak, grilled (no visible fat); baked potato; salad (no mayonnaise)
- Chilli con carne and rice
- Carvery meal of lean meat and boiled potatoes with unlimited vegetables
- Scampi Provençal
- Salmon steak; new potatoes; peas; 1 tablespoon Hollandaise sauce
- Spaghetti Napolitana
- Calves liver; potatoes; green beans
- Cannelloni
- Chinese beef and peppers or chicken and beansprouts; half portion boiled rice

▲▲▲▲▲▲▲▲▲▲▲▲

- Chicken tikka with boiled rice
- Spaghetti Bolognese
- Spaghetti marinara

- Tagliatelle with vegetables
- Vegetable curry with half portion rice and 2 tablespoons dahl
- Ravioli
- Coq au vin
- Carvery roast including 2 chunks roast potato

Desserts
(Count these as Red Extras)

▲▲

- Fresh fruit salad or figs or lychees or mango
- Sorbet

▲▲▲

- Ice cream
- Meringue with fruit topping

▲▲▲▲

- Crème caramel
- Banana split
- Strawberries and cream

▲▲▲▲▲▲

- Fruit pie (single crust) or crumble
- Pavlova
- Chocolate mousse
- Trifle
- Lemon meringue pie
- Pancakes with maple syrup
- Gâteau

RECIPES

($\triangle$ = ½ triangle)

COLD DISHES

LIGHT MAYONNAISE

(Makes 8 level tablespoons at $\triangle$ per tablespoon)

50 ml (2 fl oz) natural low-fat yogurt
40 ml (1½ fl oz) reduced-calorie mayonnaise
2 tsp fresh lemon juice
1 level tsp dry mustard powder
Salt and black pepper

Blend all the ingredients together in a small bowl; store in a covered container in fridge. Will keep for a week or more.

Variations
- Add tomato purée for seafood dressing
- Add a little curry powder for Coronation Chicken dressing
- Add fresh herbs or garlic for stronger taste
- Low-fat Bio yogurt gives a creamier result in this dressing than most ordinary low-fat natural yogurts

LIGHT COLESLAW

(Makes 2 large servings of ▲$\triangle$ each)

110 g (4 oz) white cabbage, thinly sliced and chopped
1 medium carrot, grated
25 g (1 oz) onion *or* 2 large spring onions, finely chopped
15 g (½ oz) sultanas
3 level tbsp Light Mayonnaise (see recipe above)

Combine all the ingredients well in a bowl and store in a covered container in fridge. Will keep for a few days.

Variations
- Use 25 g (1 oz) chopped dried apricots instead of the sultanas
- Use red and white cabbage instead of all white

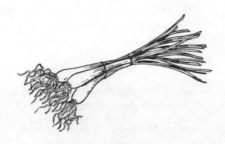

SALADE NIÇOISE
(Serves 2, ▲▲▲▲ per portion)

1 small head soft lettuce
200 g (7 oz) tinned tuna in brine, drained
50 g (2 oz) lightly cooked green beans
100 g (3½ oz) cooked potato
2 tomatoes
4 spring onions
25 g (1 oz) [good handful] watercress
4 tbsp oil-free French dressing
1 medium egg, hard-boiled and quartered
4 stoned black olives

Remove outer leaves of lettuce, then wash and tear them into pieces (discarding any that are poor). Cut the heart into four wedges and put all the lettuce into a salad bowl. Break up tuna and add to lettuce. Roughly chop the beans, potato, tomatoes, spring onions and watercress and add to bowl. Toss the salad in the oil-free dressing, then garnish with the egg and the olives.

HAWAIIAN RICE SALAD WITH CHICKEN

(Serves 2, ▲▲▲▲▲▲ per portion)

100 g (3¹/₂ oz) [dry weight] long-grain rice
or 275 g (10 oz) [cooked weight] long-grain rice
¹/₂ tsp ground turmeric
4 tbsp oil-free French dressing
100 g (3¹/₂ oz) cooked chopped chicken (no skin or bone)
1 ring pineapple, chopped
¹/₂ green pepper, de-seeded and sliced
1 stick celery, chopped
¹/₂ banana, sliced
25 g (1 oz) fresh beansprouts
¹/₂ red apple, chopped

Cook the rice, if necessary, and cool. Beat the turmeric into the dressing. Combine all the ingredients in a salad bowl.

Variation
● Vegetarians could use 100 g (3¹/₂ oz) [cooked weight] chick peas instead of the chicken

PASTA SALAD WITH CRISPY BACON

(Serves 2, ▲▲▲▲▲▲▲▲ per portion)

110 g (4 oz) [dry weight] pasta shapes of your choice
2 rashers lean-trimmed back bacon
¹/₂ red apple, chopped
1 small or ¹/₂ large ripe avocado, stoned, peeled and chopped
4 tbsp oil-free French dressing
20 g (³/₄ oz) ready-made croutons

Boil the pasta in plenty of salted water until tender (about 10 minutes). Grill the bacon rashers until crisp. Toss the apple and avocado in the dressing to prevent browning. Combine the pasta, apple, avocado and dressing in a salad bowl, crumble the bacon over and sprinkle the croutons on top.

PRAWN AND PASTA SALAD

(Serves 2, ▲▲▲▲▲▲▲▲▲▲ *per portion)*

150 g (5¹/₂ oz) [dry weight] pasta shapes of your choice
2 tbsp 1000 Island-style dressing (e.g., Kraft)
2 tbsp natural low-fat yogurt
Salt and pepper to taste
175 g (6 oz) peeled prawns
100 g (3¹/₂ oz) pineapple pieces
1 small green pepper, de-seeded and chopped
25 g (1 oz) flaked toasted almonds
Chopped parsley

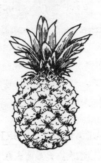

Cook the pasta in boiling salted water until tender (about 10 minutes), rinse under cold water and drain. Combine the dressing and yogurt with seasoning and any pineapple juice. Arrange the pasta, prawns, pineapple, pepper and almonds in salad bowl and toss with the dressing. Garnish with chopped parsley.

Variations
- Use melon chunks instead of the pineapple, in which case the calorie count will be a little lower
- Vegetarians could use 50 g (2 oz) Edam or 65 g (2¹/₂ oz) reduced-fat Cheddar instead of the prawns

RICE AND BEAN SALAD

(Serves 2, ▲▲▲▲▲▲▲▲▲ per portion)

This is good for using up leftover cooked rice and fridge odd-
ments.

110 g (4 oz) [dry weight] brown rice
or 275 g (10 oz) [cooked weight] brown rice
100 g (3 ½ oz) [cooked weight] brown or green lentils*
4 tbsp oil-free French dressing
1 tsp curry powder
Chopped parsley or mint
Pinch caster sugar
50 g (2 oz) red kidney beans
1 small red pepper, de-seeded and chopped
50 g (2 oz) sultanas
50 g (2 oz) mushrooms, sliced
1 small orange, peeled and chopped
25 g (1 oz) cooked sweetcorn
Lettuce leaves

Cook the rice and lentils, if necessary; drain and cool. Combine
the dressing, curry powder, herbs and sugar. Combine all the
dry ingredients except the lettuce. Arrange the lettuce in the
serving bowl and pile the rice salad into the centre.

Variations
- Use flageolet or cannellini beans instead of the kidney
  beans
- Use chopped dates instead of the sultanas
- Use white rice instead of brown, if preferred

* *To cook lentils or split peas: cover with water, bring to the
boil and simmer for 30-50 minutes until tender. Drain and use
as required.*

HOT DISHES

RATATOUILLE
(Serves 2, ▲▲ per portion)

2 tsp olive oil
1 medium onion, sliced
1 clove garlic, crushed
2 medium courgettes, sliced
1 small-to-medium aubergine, cubed
1 medium green pepper, de-seeded and chopped
4 tinned tomatoes and their juice
2 tsp chopped oregano
Salt and pepper

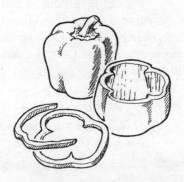

Heat the oil in a heavy-based, lidded saucepan or flameproof casserole and sauté the onion and garlic until soft, stirring frequently.

Add the rest of the ingredients and stir on a hot hob for a minute or two; then turn down the heat, cover, and simmer very gently for 1 hour. If the ratatouille looks dry towards the end of the cooking time, add some tomato juice or water.

TANGY TOMATO SOUP

(Serves 2, ▲▲ per portion)

400 g (14 oz) tinned chopped tomatoes
or 450 g (1 lb) fresh ripe tomatoes, skinned,
de-seeded and chopped
1 medium carrot, finely chopped
1 stick celery, finely chopped
1 medium onion, finely chopped
1 small red pepper, de-seeded and finely chopped (optional)
Dash of orange juice
Pinch of sugar
Pinch of ground coriander
Salt and pepper
50 ml (2 fl oz) passata
2 level tbsp fromage frais

Simmer all the ingredients, except the fromage frais, together in
a covered saucepan until the vegetables are tender. Purée in a
blender, return the mixture to the pan and reheat. Check seasoning. Serve with the fromage frais swirled on the top.

NEW-STYLE ROAST POTATOES

*(Makes 400 g [14 oz], ▲▲▲▲▲▲▲▲▲ for the whole quantity,
▲▲ per 100 g [3¹/₂ oz])*

375 g (13 oz) new or small waxy potatoes
2 tsp olive oil
1 tbsp lemon juice
1 tbsp chopped fresh thyme
1 tsp finely chopped garlic
Little coarse sea salt and coarsely ground black pepper

Preheat oven to 400°F/200°C/Gas mark 6.
　Scrub the potatoes, leaving the peel on. Cut them into smallish pieces of about 25 g (1 oz) each, if necessary (if very small,

leave whole). Pat dry on kitchen paper and place in a roasting pan of suitable size (not too big).

Drizzle the oil and lemon juice over, then sprinkle with the thyme, garlic, salt and pepper, and, using your hands, make sure each potato is well coated with the oil and seasonings. If you can leave the potatoes to absorb the flavours for a while, so much the better.

Place in preheated oven and roast for 50 minutes, turning once, until golden and cooked through.

CHICKEN SALSA TACOS

(Serves 2, ▲▲▲▲▲▲ per portion)

175 g (6 oz) cooked chopped chicken (no skin)
25 g (1 oz) red kidney beans, chopped
2 medium ripe tomatoes, finely chopped
4 large spring onions, finely chopped
2 tsp corn oil
1 small green pepper, finely chopped
2 tsp lime juice
1 level tsp Mexican seasoning (or chilli powder) to taste
1 level tsp cornflour
1/2 tsp ground cumin
50 ml (2 fl oz) passata
4 taco shells
Fresh coriander or lettuce, chopped

Simmer all the ingredients, except the tacos and coriander/lettuce, in a small covered pan for 20-30 minutes. Heat the tacos in the oven; fill with mixture, garnish with coriander/lettuce and serve.

Variation
● The filling can also be used for pancakes, or over rice, pasta or baked potatoes

RICE-STUFFED BAKED VEGETABLES

(Serves 2, ▲▲▲▲▲▲ per portion)

75 g (3 oz) [dry weight] long-grain rice
or 200 g (7 oz) [ready-cooked weight] rice
2 medium aubergines
200 g (7 oz) chopped tomatoes with herbs
15 g (½ oz) chopped almonds or pine nuts
1 tbsp tomato purée
2 large spring onions, finely chopped
1 clove garlic, chopped
Salt and pepper
Passata and water (approx. 275 ml, 10 fl oz)
or tomato juice
100 g (3½ oz) tuna in brine, drained,
or pre-cooked brown lentils *or* 75 g (3 oz) lean chopped ham
1 level tbsp grated Parmesan cheese
1 tbsp chopped parsley

Cook the rice if necessary. Halve the aubergines and scoop out about half of the flesh. Chop and reserve this flesh. Add the aubergines halves to a large pan of boiling salted water and blanch for 3 minutes. Drain and pat dry.

In a saucepan, simmer the rice, aubergine flesh, tomatoes, almonds/pine nuts, tomato purée, onions, garlic, seasoning and a little passata for 10 minutes. Add the flaked tuna, lentils or ham. Place the aubergine halves in a shallow baking dish and fill with the rice mixture. Pour the passata mixed with water (or tomato juice) around the aubergines at the base of the dish. Cover with foil or a lid and bake at 400°F/200°C/Gas mark 6 for 1 hour or until aubergines are tender. Sprinkle the Parmesan and parsley over to serve.

Variations
● You could use large courgettes or de-seeded peppers instead of the aubergines and treat them in exactly the same way

- You can also use large tomatoes or mushrooms, but don't blanch tomatoes or mushrooms and be sure to reduce the cooking time

ITALIAN-STYLE ROAST VEGETABLES
with accompaniment
(Serves 2, ▲▲▲▲▲▲ *per portion)*

1 beef tomato, cut into 4 thick slices
4 large open-cup mushrooms
1 yellow pepper, de-seeded and quartered
1 small aubergine, cut into 2 cm slices
1 red onion, cut crossways into 4 slices
1 tbsp olive oil
Salt and pepper
1 clove garlic, chopped
75 g (3 oz) [dry weight] bulgar wheat
or brown rice *or* 50 g (2 oz) crusty bread
1 tbsp stoned black olives, chopped
1 tbsp sun-dried tomatoes, drained on kitchen paper
and chopped
Chopped thyme and parsley
4 tsp balsamic vinegar
1 tsp grated Parmesan cheese

Line a roasting pan with foil and place the prepared fresh vegetables on it. Put the olive oil into a saucer and, using a pastry brush, brush the oil over the vegetables. Sprinkle some salt, black pepper and garlic on the top. Roast for 20-30 minutes or until the vegetables are well browned and soft throughout. Meanwhile, soak the bulgar wheat or cook the rice and keep it warm. Serve the vegetables with the olives, sun-dried tomatoes, herbs, vinegar, any remaining olive oil, and Parmesan cheese sprinkled over, alongside the wheat or rice or bread.

Variations
- You can try other vegetables, such as globe artichokes or courgettes, cooked this way
- You can also try grilling them for a slightly different result, or, of course, barbecuing

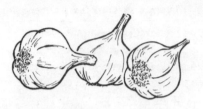

INDONESIAN STIR-FRY

(Serves 2, ▲▲▲▲▲▲ per portion)

65 g (2½ oz) [dry weight] fragrant rice
2 tsp corn oil
100 g (3½ oz) turkey or chicken (no skin),
cut into small strips
8 baby sweetcorns
1 carrot, cut into thin strips
100 g (3½ oz) fresh beansprouts
1 red pepper, de-seeded and finely chopped
50 g (2 oz) peeled prawns
4 spring onions, chopped
1 clove garlic, crushed
1 tbsp light soya sauce
1 tsp 7-Spice seasoning
Pinch of sugar
2 tbsp (or as necessary) chicken stock

Cook the rice in boiling salted water until tender; rinse in colander and set aside.

Heat the oil in a non-stick pan and stir-fry the poultry and sweetcorn until the meat is lightly golden. Add the rest of the ingredients and stir-fry for further 3 minutes. Add the drained rice and stir for 1 minute. Extra chicken stock can be added at any time if the mixture looks too dry or if it sticks.

CHINESE BEEF AND RED PEPPER STIR-FRY

(Serves 2, ▲▲▲▲▲▲ per portion)

65 g (2½ oz) [dry weight] egg thread noodles
2 tsp corn or sesame oil
125 g (4½ oz) lean beef steak, cut into strips
1 large red pepper, de-seeded and cut into large thick strips
6 spring onions, cut in half lengthways
50 g (2 oz) beansprouts
2 tbsp sweetcorn
1 tbsp oyster sauce
2 tsp light soya sauce
50 ml (2 fl oz) beef stock

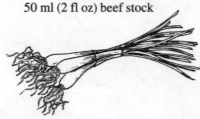

Soak the noodles according to the pack instructions (usually about 5 minutes).

Head the oil in a non-stick wok or frying pan and stir-fry the beef, red pepper and onion until the beef is brown (about 3 minutes). Add the rest of the ingredients, turn the heat down and stir-fry for 1 minute. Add the noodles to the pan, with a little more beef stock if necessary, stir and serve.

Variation
● You can serve the Beef Stir-Fry with boiled rice instead of noodles if you prefer. In that case, don't add the rice to the frying pan but serve it separately, precooked

TOMATO SAUCE

(Makes 4 servings of ▲△ each.
Freeze what you don't need)

1 tbsp olive oil
1 onion, finely chopped
Dash of white wine
400 g (14 oz) tinned chopped tomatoes
1 tsp Worcester sauce
1 clove garlic, crushed
1 tsp brown sugar
1 tbsp tomato purée
1 tsp chopped basil
Salt and black pepper

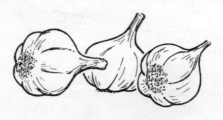

Heat the oil in a saucepan, add the onion and stir until soft. Add the rest of the ingredients and stir and simmer for 20 minutes until you have a rich sauce. Check seasoning. For a smoother result, press the sauce through a sieve.

Variations
- Add chopped and de-seeded red chilli for a hot sauce
- Add sliced black olives for a quick Italian pasta sauce

CAULIFLOWER AND BACON GRATIN

(Serves 2, ▲▲▲▲▲▲ per portion)

2 slices lean back bacon, trimmed of fat
1 small-to-medium (approx. 275 g [10 oz]
prepared weight) cauliflower, cut into florets
75 g (3 oz) whole green beans, cut into 2 cm (1 inch) pieces
1 quantity (2 portions) Cheese Sauce (see following recipe)
15 g (½ oz) reduced-fat Cheddar cheese, grated
25 g (1 oz) brown breadcrumbs

Grill the bacon until crisp, then crumble it. Boil or microwave the cauliflower and beans until barely tender and arrange in two gratin dishes with the bacon scattered over. Pour on top the cheese sauce, scatter over the extra cheese and breadcrumbs and grill until golden.

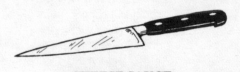

CHEESE SAUCE

(Serves 2, ▲▲▲ per portion)

15 g (½ oz) low-fat spread
15 g (½ oz) plain flour
175 ml (6 fl oz) skimmed milk at room temperature
30 g (1 ¼ oz) reduced-fat Cheddar cheese, grated
Salt and pepper to taste

Melt the low-fat spread in a saucepan, add the flour and cook, stirring, for a minute. Slowly add the milk and stir until the consistency is thick. Add the cheese and seasoning and stir until the cheese melts. Check for seasoning.

This cheese sauce can be used in all kinds of savoury dishes – e.g., over pancakes, with plain fish or to top moussaka and lasagne.

JAMBALAYA

(Serves 2, ▲▲▲▲▲▲▲▲ per portion)

2 tsp corn oil
1 boneless chicken breast (approx. 110 g [4 oz]),
cut into small cubes
110 g (4 oz) pork fillet, cut into small cubes
1 small onion, very finely chopped
4 spring onions, chopped
1 stick celery, chopped
1 tsp Cajun seasoning
1 clove garlic, chopped
110 g (4 oz) [dry weight] long-grain rice,
boiled and drained
2 tomatoes, skinned and chopped
50 ml (2 fl oz) chicken stock
Salt and pepper
1 tbsp fresh chopped parsley

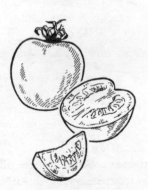

Heat the oil in a non-stick frying pan and fry the chicken, pork,
onion and spring onion on a hot hob, stirring frequently. Turn
the heat down and add the rest of the ingredients. Cook for 5
minutes, stirring frequently. Check for seasoning and serve.

SEAFOOD TAGLIATELLE

(Serves 2, ▲▲▲▲▲▲▲▲▲ per portion)

125 g (4 ½ oz) [dry weight] tagliatelle
2 tsp olive oil
1 small onion, very finely chopped
1 clove garlic, crushed
Pinch of saffron powder
2 tbsp dry white wine
50 g (2 oz) broccoli florets
25 g (1 oz) petit pois
50 g (2 oz) button mushrooms, sliced
80 g (3 ¼ oz) peeled prawns
4 crab sticks, thawed and chopped
25 g (1 oz) shelled mussels (thawed if frozen)
2 tsp lemon juice
2 tbsp skimmed milk
Salt and pepper
2 tbsp extra-thick single cream
or reduced-calorie double cream

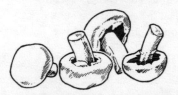

Cook the tagliatelle in boiling salted water for 10 minutes or until it is just soft. Drain in colander.

While the pasta is cooking, heat the oil in a non-stick frying pan and stir-fry the onion until soft. Add the garlic, saffron and wine and allow the mixture to bubble for a minute. Add the broccoli, peas and mushrooms and stir for 2 minutes. Add all the seafood, lemon juice and milk and simmer for 2-3 minutes until the fish is heated through. Add the seasoning and cream, stir, check the seasoning, and serve over the drained pasta.

SPICED PORK WITH RICE

(Serves 2, ▲▲▲▲▲▲▲▲▲ *per portion)*

125 g (4 ½ oz) [dry weight] ready-mixed
long-grain and wild rice
2 tsp corn oil
1 small red pepper, de-seeded
and finely chopped
1 small onion, finely chopped
140 g (5 oz) pork fillet, cubed
1 heaped tsp garam masala (or to taste)
110 g (4 oz) button mushrooms, halved
1 tsp French mustard
50 ml (2 fl oz) chicken stock
2 tsp lemon juice
Salt and pepper
2 heaped tbsp Greek yogurt or sour cream
Chopped fresh coriander or parsley

Boil the rice according to the packet instructions (usually about
20 minutes). Drain when wild rice is tender.

Meanwhile, heat the oil in a non-stick frying pan and fry the
red pepper and onion until soft, stirring. Set to one side of the
pan and add the pork. Cook over high heat, turning the pork
cubes until they are brown on all sides. Turn the heat down, add
the garam masala and stir. Add the mushrooms, mustard, stock,
lemon juice and seasoning and simmer on Low for 5 minutes.
When pork is tender, add yogurt or sour cream, stir and bring
gently to simmer. Serve immediately over the rice, garnished
with the coriander/parsley.

Variations
- You can use chicken fillet in this recipe, too
- Alternatively, try the basic recipe but use Hungarian paprika
  instead of the garam masala

SWEET AND SOUR STIR-FRY

(Serves 2, ▲▲▲▲▲▲▲▲▲ per portion)

110 g (4 oz) [dry weight] long-grain rice
or egg thread noodles
2 tsp corn oil
1 medium carrot, cut into matchsticks
1 small red pepper, de-seeded and sliced
50 g (2 oz) small broccoli florets
50 g (2 oz) baby sweetcorn cobs
50 g (2 oz) green beans, halved
50 g (2 oz) tinned bamboo shoots
4 spring onions, halved lengthways
3 Chinese leaves, sliced
75 g (3 oz) mushrooms, sliced
15 g (½ oz) flaked almonds

Sweet-and-Sour Sauce
1 rounded tsp cornflour
1 level tbsp runny honey
50 ml (2 fl oz) orange juice
1 tbsp light soya sauce
1½ tbsp white-wine vinegar
1 tbsp white wine
2 tsp tomato purée

Mix all the sauce ingredients together in a bowl and set aside. If using rice, put it on the boil, or soak the noodles and set aside.

Heat the oil in a non-stick frying pan or wok. Stir-fry the carrot, red pepper, broccoli, sweetcorn and green beans for 3 minutes. Add the bamboo shoots, spring onions, Chinese leaves and mushrooms and stir again for 1 minute. Add the almonds and the sweet-and-sour sauce and stir for 1 minute or until sauce has thickened. If using noodles, add to the wok to reheat for a few seconds. If using rice, serve the sweet-and-sour vegetables over the rice.

Variation

- Use 100 g (3½ oz) firm white cubed fish instead of the almonds, or you could use firm tofu. In either case, add it to the pan with the first batch of vegetables

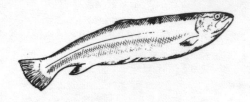

SEAFOOD CRUMBLE

(Serves 2, ▲▲▲▲▲▲ per portion)

100 g (3½ oz) broccoli florets
275 g (10 oz) cod or other white fish fillet
25 g (1 oz) peeled prawns
75 g (3 oz) button mushrooms, halved
4 spring onions, chopped
100 g (3½ oz) Greek yogurt
2 tbsp skimmed milk
2 tsp lemon juice
1 tsp cornflour
Salt and pepper
1 tbsp chopped parsley
1 tsp chopped dill
1 clove garlic, crushed
40 g (1½ oz) reduced-fat Cheddar cheese, grated
25 g (1 oz) brown breadcrumbs

Boil the broccoli until just soft, drain and reserve. Poach or microwave the fish until just cooked and flake it into 2 individual gratin dishes. Add the broccoli, prawns, raw mushrooms and onion to the dishes, dividing equally. In a bowl, mix together the yogurt, milk, lemon juice, cornflour, salt, pepper, parsley, dill, garlic and half the cheese until well combined. Pour the mixture over the fish and vegetables. Top with the breadcrumbs and remaining cheese and bake at 400°F/200°C/Gas mark 6 until the top is golden (about 20 minutes).

BEEF AND VEGETABLE CURRY WITH RICE

(Serves 2, ▲▲▲▲▲▲▲▲▲▲ per portion)

2 tsp corn oil
1 onion, chopped
175 g (6 oz) extra-lean braising beef, cubed
1 clove garlic, crushed
2 tsp curry powder (or to taste)
75 g (3 oz) potato, parboiled and cubed
100 g (3½ oz) cauliflower florets
or aubergine, cubed
50 g (2 oz) green beans
200 g (7 oz) tinned chopped tomatoes
1 tbsp tomato purée
40 g (1½ oz) [dry weight] brown, green or red lentils
or split peas
Pinch of brown sugar
110 ml (4 fl oz) beef stock
Salt
100 g (3½ oz) [dry weight] long-grain rice

Heat the oil in a non-stick pan and fry the onion until soft. Add the beef and fry till brown. Turn the heat down and add the garlic and curry powder; stir for 1 minute. Add the potato, cauliflower, beans, tomatoes, tomato purée, lentils, sugar and beef stock. Cover and simmer for 1 hour or until everything is tender. (Check after approx. 45 minutes that the curry isn't drying out; if it is, add a little water or beef stock.) Add salt to taste. Meanwhile, boil the rice and serve with the curry.

VEGETABLE LASAGNE

(Serves 2, ▲▲▲▲▲▲▲▲▲▲▲ *per portion)*

2 tsp olive oil
1 small onion, finely chopped
1 large courgette, sliced
1 small aubergine, sliced
1 small red or green pepper, de-seeded and chopped
75 g (3 oz) [dry weight] green or brown lentils
300 ml (11 fl oz) vegetable stock made with cube
200 g (7 oz) tinned chopped tomatoes
1 level tbsp tomato purée
1/2 tsp ground coriander
1 tsp oregano
Salt and pepper
4 sheets 'no-precook' lasagne
1 portion Cheese Sauce (see recipe on page 205)
2 tbsp Parmesan cheese

Heat the oil in a non-stick pan and stir-fry the onion until soft. Add the courgette, aubergine and pepper and stir-fry for 1 minute. Add the lentils, stock, tomatoes, tomato purée, herbs and seasoning. Stir, cover and simmer gently for 40-50 minutes until the vegetables and lentils are tender and the sauce is rich but quite runny (this is because the lasagne sheets absorb liquid). If the sauce is too thick, add a little water or stock. In 2 individual lasagne dishes (or a suitable shallow baking dish) put half the vegetable mixture in the base and cover each with a lasagne sheet. Cover with the remaining vegetable mix and remaining lasagne sheets, top with the cheese sauce to cover completely, then sprinkle the grated cheese over. Bake at 375°F/190°C/Gas mark 5 until the top is golden and bubbling (about 25 minutes).

Variation
- Try precooked haricot beans instead of the lentils – in which case, reduce the quantity of stock to approx. 200 ml (7 fl oz)

PASTA SPIRALS WITH MINCED BEEF
AND VEGETABLES
(Serves 2, ▲▲▲▲▲▲▲▲▲▲▲▲ *per portion)*

1 quantity (2 portions) Basic Minced Beef
(see following recipe)
200 g (7 oz) tinned chopped tomatoes
50 g (2 oz) sweetcorn *or* tinned borlotti beans, drained
25 g (1 oz) petit pois
50 g (2 oz) green beans, cut into 2 cm pieces
125 g (4½ oz) [dry weight] tricolour pasta spirals
2 tsp Parmesan cheese

Mix the minced beef with all the vegetables and simmer in a pan for 10 minutes while you cook the pasta in boiling salted water. Serve the beef and vegetables tossed with the spirals and sprinkled with the Parmesan cheese.

BASIC MINCED BEEF
(Serves 2, ▲▲▲▲ *per portion)*

Enough corn oil to brush on a non-stick frying pan
(or use Fry Light spray)
175 g (6 oz) extra-lean minced beef
1 medium onion, finely chopped
1 stick celery, finely chopped
1 small carrot, finely chopped
150 ml (5½ fl oz) beef stock made with cube
1 tbsp tomato purée
1 tsp Mediterranean herbs
1 tsp Worcester sauce
Salt and black pepper

Coat the non-stick pan with the oil and heat gently. Add the mince and brown it over a medium heat, stirring from time to time. Remove the mince with a slatted spoon when well browned, leaving any fat which has run from the meat. In this fat, stir-fry the onion until soft (about 5 minutes). Add the celery and carrot and 1 tablespoon of the stock, and stir again for a few minutes. Return the mince to the pan and add the rest of the ingredients. Stir well and simmer for 20 minutes or until you have a rich minced beef sauce.

Variations

● This basic minced beef can be used for all kinds of dishes – e.g., cottage pie, or to fill a filo pie, or with the addition of some garlic and a dash of wine it makes a good Bolognese sauce

● Mixed with rice, it's a good stuffed vegetable filling, or try it in pancakes topped with Cheese Sauce (see recipe on page 205)

CHILLI CON CARNE AND RICE

(Serves 2, ▲▲▲▲▲▲▲▲▲▲ *per portion)*

1 large green pepper, de-seeded and chopped
150 g (5½ oz) [drained weight] tinned red kidney beans
200 g (7 oz) tinned chopped tomatoes
1 tsp chilli powder (or to taste),
or 1 whole fresh chilli, chopped
1 portion Basic Minced Beef (see preceding recipe)
110 g (4 oz) [dry weight] long-grain rice

Mix the green pepper, beans, tomato and chilli into the minced beef and simmer in a pan for 20 minutes while you cook the rice. Serve the chilli with the rice.

Variations

● Fresh chillis are widely available now and often have a better flavour than dried powder, but unless you like your chilli very hot, remove the seeds before chopping the chilli. You can also use dried whole chilies, for which the same applies

- TVP or VegeMince can be used instead of beef mince in all these recipes based on mince
- Try black-eye beans or borlotti beans in your chilli

CHICKEN AND MUSHROOM RISOTTO

(Serves 2, ▲▲▲▲▲▲▲▲▲▲ per portion)

1 tbsp olive oil *or* 15 g (½ oz)butter
1 smallish onion, finely chopped
110 g (4 oz) lean chicken fillet,
chopped into small cubes
175 g (6 oz) [dry weight] risotto rice
Dash of dry wine
500 ml (18 fl oz) chicken stock
25 g (1 oz) lean ham, cut into small strips
175 g (6 oz) mushrooms
(preferably at least two kinds),
sliced or torn
25 g (1 oz) petit pois
1 tsp chopped basil
A little salt to taste (optional)
Black pepper

Heat the oil in a non-stick frying pan and fry the onion until soft. Add the chicken and stir until tinged gold. Add the rice and stir for 1 minute. Add the wine and bring to bubbling. Add two-thirds of the stock, ham, mushrooms, peas, basil and seasoning, and stir the mixture; simmer gently, stirring from time to time. Add more stock as necessary. The risotto is cooked when most of the stock is absorbed and the rice is tender and creamy.

Variation
- Vegetarians can omit the chicken, use vegetable stock and top the risotto with 3 tablespoons of Parmesan cheese

LUXURY PAELLA

(Serves 2, ▲▲▲▲▲▲▲▲▲▲▲▲▲ per portion)

6 giant prawns
or 75 g (3 oz) peeled prawns
8 mussels, fresh in shells
or 12 frozen mussels, thawed
1½ tbsp olive oil
100 g (3½ oz) chicken or pork fillet,
cut into bite-sized cubes
1 small onion, chopped
1 small red pepper, de-seeded and chopped
Approx. 550 ml (1 pint) chicken or fish stock
1 clove garlic, crushed
1 sachet saffron
Pinch of paprika
150 g (5½ oz) [dry weight] long-grain rice
1 large tomato, chopped
25 g (1 oz) peas
100 g (3½ oz) firm white fish
(e.g., monkfish, swordfish or cod)
4 cooked or tinned artichoke hearts
1 tbsp chopped parsley
Salt and pepper

If peeling the prawns yourself, leave the tails on. If necessary,
prepare the fresh mussels.

Heat the oil in a paella pan or a large frying pan and fry the
chicken or pork until golden. Remove with a slatted spoon and
set aside. Add the onion and red pepper to the pan and fry until
soft. Add the stock, garlic, saffron and paprika, return the chick-
en/pork to the pan, bring to the boil and then turn down the heat.
Simmer for 5 minutes, add the rice, tomato and peas and simmer
gently for 15 minutes or so, adding more stock if the rice dries out
before it is tender, and stirring from time to time. When the rice is

nearly tender, add the white fish, prawns, mussels, artichoke hearts and parsley. Season and simmer for 5 minutes and serve.

(**Note:** The rice grains should be tender but not mushy – paella is a little drier than risotto. If using fresh mussels in their shells, discard any that have not opened when ready to serve.)

PASTA AND TUNA BAKE

(Serves 2, ▲▲▲▲▲▲▲▲▲▲ *per portion)*

125 g (4¹/₂ oz) [dry weight] pasta shapes (e.g., macaroni)
175 g (6 oz) tuna in brine, drained
1 tbsp chopped parsley
2 black olives, stoned and chopped (optional)
2 tomatoes, skinned, de-seeded and chopped
2 spring onions, finely chopped
1 quantity (2 portions) Cheese Sauce (see recipe on page 205)
25 g (1 oz) brown breadcrumbs
25 g (1 oz) reduced-fat Cheddar cheese, grated
Little salt if necessary

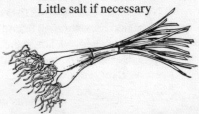

Boil the pasta until just tender (about 10 minutes); drain and keep warm. Arrange the tuna, pasta, parsley, olives, tomato and onion in 2 gratin dishes (or 1 baking dish if preferred) and pour sauce over. Top with the breadcrumbs and cheese and bake at 400°F/200°C/Gas mark 6 for 20 minutes until top is golden.

Variation
- Use 100 g (3¹/₂ oz) pasta and 25 g (1 oz) cooked cannellini (white Italian) beans or butter beans

DESSERTS

FRUIT-FILLED FLANS

(Serves 2, ▲▲▲▲ *per portion)*

2 tsp sunflower oil or use Fry Light spray
2 oblong sheets filo pastry (thawed if frozen)
1 kiwifruit or small peach
1 small banana
50 g (2 oz) grapes or strawberries, halved
1 small orange
Dash of lemon juice
50 ml (2 fl oz) orange juice
1 tsp arrowroot
2 tsp low-sugar apricot jam
4 tsp Greek yogurt

Preheat oven to 400°F/200°C/Gas mark 6. Brush or spray 2 individual flan tins or foil pudding tins with oil very lightly.

Cut the sheets of filo into four each and layer them together, trimming the edges into a rough round. Brush the top layer with oil or spray as before. Line the two containers with the filo layers and press in gently. Bake for a few minutes until golden brown. Remove from oven, leave them to cool, then remove from containers.

Meanwhile prepare the fruit by peeling, deseeding and chopping as necessary into bite-sized pieces. Toss the banana pieces in the lemon juice to prevent them browning. Mix the orange juice, arrowroot and jam together and heat in a small saucepan until the mixture becomes a sauce. Arrange the fruit in the filo cases and pour the sauce over. Top each with the yogurt to serve.

Variation
● Substitute other fruit according to your preference and what is in season

FRUIT PANCAKES WITH CREAMY SAUCE

(Serves 2, ▲▲▲ per portion)

Pancakes (makes 2)
40 g (1½ oz) plain flour
½ size-3 egg, beaten
40 ml (1½ fl oz) skimmed milk mixed with
25 ml (1 fl oz) water
Salt
1 tsp oil *or* Fry Light spray to coat frying pan

Fruit filling
75 g (3 oz) strawberries, sliced, *or* raspberries
50 g (2 oz) peach, sliced, *or* kiwifruit, sliced
1 tsp fructose

Topping
3 tbsp fromage frais
1 tbsp skimmed milk
1 tsp fructose
or
3 tbsp Greek yogurt

Prepare the fruit filling by mixing the fruit with the fructose and leave in fridge until needed. Prepare the topping by mixing together the fromage frais, milk and fructose and leave in fridge until needed.

To make the pancakes, beat together in a small mixing bowl the flour, egg, skimmed milk mixture and salt until smooth. Brush a small non-stick frying pan with the oil, or spray it with Fry Light, and heat the pan until very hot. Add half the pancake mixture, swirling it around to coat evenly. Cook the pancake on high heat until golden on the underside. With a large spatula, turn the pancake over and cook the other side for a few seconds.

Turn out on to a warmed serving plate, fill with the fruit mixture and fold or roll up. Top with the topping or the Greek yogurtand serve.

(**Note:** If you are cooking for two and don't want to waste half
an egg, make up double the quantity of pancake mixture and
freeze half either as batter or as the made-up pancakes.)

BLACKCURRANT CHEESECAKE

(Serves 8, ▲▲▲ per portion)

40 g (1½ oz) low-fat spread
8 digestive biscuits, crushed
300 g (11 oz) blackcurrants, topped and tailed
1 rounded tbsp fructose
300 g (11 oz) fromage frais
1 tsp lemon juice
1½ sachets of gelatine
150 ml (5½ fl oz) low-fat Bio yogurt

Melt the low-fat spread and mix the crushed biscuits into it in a
bowl. Press the biscuit mixture firmly into the base of a 7-inch
(18 cm), loose-bottomed cake tin.

Simmer the blackcurrants with a very little water for a few
minutes, then stir in the fructose. Whiz the blackcurrants, fromage frais and lemon juice in a blender. Dissolve the gelatine in
a little very hot water and stir it and the yogurt very thoroughly
into the blackcurrant mixture. Spoon the mixture evenly over
the biscuit base. Chill until set.

Variation
● Try using strawberries instead of blackcurrants

THE FREESTYLE PLAN

For long-term slimming, you can use the pyramid below and the appendix at the back of the book to devise meals and recipes of your own.

All you do is make up your day's diet aiming, as near as possible, for these triangles: **9 Starch, 7 Fruit and Vegetable, 5 Protein, 3 Fat,** and **1 Sugar and Alcohol.**

The foods in the appendix are listed together in these groups to make life easier, and you can read Step Six for more information on building a programme from these lists.

I suggest that to start with you draw up some blank triangles like this one below and cross off the triangles in each level as you eat the food they represent. The total number of triangles in this pyramid is 25, giving you a daily total of approximately 1,250 calories. If this amount is too little for you, you can always add extra triangles, but try to keep them in proportion so you retain the pyramid shape to your diet.

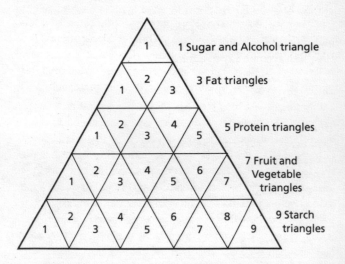

STEP FIVE
Get Moving!

One of the very best assets you have in your quest for slimness is your body's ability to move. Activity is just as vital to healthy weight loss as diet is, and yet many of us 'move' so little, that from waking in the morning to going to bed at night we barely burn up more calories (i.e., use up no more energy) than when we *are* asleep!

'How can that *be*?', I can hear you say. 'I'm busy all day long with never a moment's rest.'

I'm not disputing that, but let me illustrate what I mean, by telling you about a female acquaintance of mine who has what I would describe as the busy lifestyle, typical of the 90s woman. Here's an average day in her life:

She takes a bath, gets dressed and prepares breakfast for herself and her eight-year-old son. She drops her son off at school by car and drives on to her workplace. There she takes the lift up to her office and spends a busy morning sorting out accounts. Often she is so busy that she has a packed lunch at her desk (brought in for her by a colleague). After finishing work, she takes the lift back down to her car and stops off at the supermarket before picking her son up from the childminder's. Back home she cooks her son's tea, looks at the newspaper, reads with her son, puts some washing in the machine, puts her son to bed and then prepares her own evening meal. She spends the last two hours of the evening exhausted in front of the TV.

Yes, that's certainly a busy day – a *modern* busy day, where the brain is busy, the mind is stressed and there is never enough time ... But the *body* – the muscles, the heart and the lungs – is severely under-used, except in a negative way. And yes, this friend of mine *does* have a weight problem although she doesn't eat a lot.

Bodies are meant to be used. Yet, thanks largely to modern society and science, we have, in the main, got out of the habit of using them enough. Not only are most of us unfit, but also we are not burning up nearly as many calories as people used to, even fifty years ago – so the surplus food is stored as fat.

Why have we as a nation got so lazy? We live in a world increasingly designed to deter us from having to 'move' at all! Our work more frequently involves sitting, rather than moving or even standing. We take the car everywhere instead of walking; we use domestic appliances, instead of elbow grease, to clean everything; we use lifts or escalators, rarely stairs; we watch sport on TV instead of doing it ourselves. And we are reluctant to compensate for the inactivity of our working and domestic lives by being physically active in our leisure time.

The comprehensive Allied Dunbar National Fitness Survey of 1992 found that eight out of ten women and seven out of ten men in the UK don't even take enough exercise to keep themselves healthy. So physical activity is a habit we need to relearn, not only to help us to get, and stay, slim, but for health reasons too. Bodies that cry out for use and don't get it protest in many ways, from everyday aches and pains, sluggishness, and digestive troubles, to life-threatening problems such as heart disease. And on a very basic level, an under-used, unfit body can be an inconvenience in many aspects of everyday life. Many of us can't even run, stretch or bend to pick up from the floor.

Activity, while not quite a cure-all, is certainly a free gift we can't afford to ignore. Remember, bodies like to be used. They respond by rewarding you for being used. So don't neglect your body any longer and treat it like a discarded lawnmower or an outgrown bicycle. Those you can replace, but you can't replace your body.

Why are we so reluctant to move?

For many people, the very word 'exercise' makes them shudder! And if you are overweight you are probably one of those people. It may be that the main reason you don't take much exercise at present is because you lack motivation. And the reason you lack motivation is that you don't know how to make exercise work for you or how to make it 'user-friendly'.

In Steps One to Four, you learned and began to put into practice 'slim eating'. Now that you are beginning to feel more confident about your ability to take control of your eating habits, we can concentrate on finding the right way to get *you* moving. In the next few pages you will begin to see that it really is possible for you to increase your physical activity without it being a pain, a strain, a bore or a chore.

Motivating yourself

For most people the promise of being fitter is simply not a strong enough motivation. What you need to do is:

1. Take an overview of exercise and activity and discover all the benefits it can bring.
2. Decide which of these benefits are most appropriate to you, and therefore will help to keep you motivated.
3. Decide upon the best plan of action to obtain those benefits, taking into account your personality, lifestyle and physical needs and problems.

First, we need to understand that not all exercise has the same effect on our bodies. A daily walk, for example, will provide completely different benefits from, say, a yoga session. So the very first step to finding the right exercise strategy for you is to understand the various effects of different forms of exercise.

THE FITNESS TRIANGLE

Think of total fitness as a triangle. Each corner of the triangle is a different component of total fitness, each with its own contribution to make towards improving your wellbeing and health:

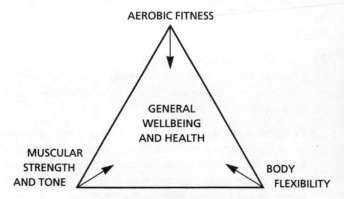

AEROBIC FITNESS

GENERAL
WELLBEING
AND HEALTH

MUSCULAR
STRENGTH
AND TONE

BODY
FLEXIBILITY

AEROBIC (HEART AND LUNG/CARDIOVASCULAR) FITNESS

The top corner of the triangle – and possibly the most important one for slimmers – is aerobic fitness, sometimes called heart and lung fitness, cardiovascular fitness or stamina.

This is what most people think of as 'fitness'. When you are not aerobically fit, you easily become breathless when walking briskly, walking uphill, running a few paces, or performing almost any sudden physical task. If you regularly exercise your heart and lungs in an 'aerobic' way, you gradually become aerobically fitter; your lungs take in more air with each breath, and your heart does its job more efficiently, pumping more blood and oxygen around the body with each beat, so that a fit heart often beats more slowly than an unfit heart.

All aerobic exercise makes your heart beat faster. Examples of aerobic training activity include: walking, jogging, cycling, swimming, aerobics classes, stepping and rowing. The fitter you become, the harder the task you will have to set yourself in order to improve your fitness still further.

There are many degrees of aerobic fitness. Not everyone needs to – or indeed can – achieve the same level. For everyday life and benefits it may be sufficient simply to increase your aerobic fitness mildly, rather than even thinking of trying to achieve levels attained by professional athletes, for instance.

The benefits of aerobic fitness

Look through the list of benefits that being fit (or fitter) aerobically can bring you, and tick which ones you would particularly like to achieve:

☐ Freedom to eat more. You can eat more while you lose weight or, in theory, lose weight slowly *without* eating less because aerobic exercise burns up more calories per session than any other form of exercise. This is because the increased oxygen uptake and effort increases your metabolic rate, not only while you are exercising but also for some time after you have stopped. Small, regular sessions can keep your metabolic rate permanently raised!

☐ Less hunger. Most people who do periods of steady aerobic exercise report better control of eating habits, including less craving for sweet, fatty foods, as well as less inclination to drink alcohol or to smoke.

☐ Increased stamina. You will have more energy to cope with everyday things like walking, pushing prams and walking uphill. If you've always lagged behind on a walk, it's brilliant for once to be the one in front shouting 'come on!'

☐ Stress relief. In many tests, aerobic exercise has been found to reduce stress levels and to induce relaxation and well-being.

☐ Reduced risk of cardiovascular (heart) disease and failure. Aerobic activity lowers blood pressure and increases the levels of the heart-protecting, high-density lipoproteins in the blood. By increasing the diameter of the coronary arteries, it also lessens the risk of 'furring' (blocked arteries). In addition, it helps the heart by helping to reduce weight and stress.

☐ Improved circulation – you feel the cold less!

☐ Less likelihood of varicose veins.

☐ Improved skin. The extra flow of oxygen and blood to your skin results in a healthy glow and a smoother skin tending to fewer spots and fewer open pores. Hair condition also benefits.

☐ Loss of body fat from all over the body. Aerobic exercise speeds up the rate at which we burn body fat. This, combined with the fact that the large muscles of the body used in the aerobic activity will become stronger and firmer, will result in a more well-defined, attractive shape.

☐ Better digestive system. The rate of digestion and elimination of food is speeded up. Aerobic activity combined with healthy eating alleviates problems such as indigestion and constipation.

☐ Improved quality of sleep. People who regularly exercise aerobically rarely need sleeping pills or have insomnia. They have sound, deep, refreshing sleep.

☐ For women, a reduction in pre-menstrual symptoms such as stomach cramps and tension.

☐ Regular aerobic activity increases bone density and lessens the risk of osteoporosis after the menopause.

☐ Enhanced powers of concentration and better brain performance all round. This is due to the increased oxygen flow to the brain.

☐ More cheerful and energetic disposition. You will feel less sluggish, depressed and lethargic. This is due partly to the increased oxygen uptake which acts like a tonic on your body and brain, and partly to the release of endorphins ('happy hormones').

☐ Better sex life and increased libido. For the same reasons outlined above.

☐ Greater mobility and wellbeing through to old age.

The good news is that if you are unfit, it doesn't take a lot to markedly improve. First try this aerobic test:

Aerobic fitness test

1. Measure out a mile (1.6 km) walk on the flat (using a car milometer or a map). Then, put on sensible shoes and comfortable clothes and warm up by marching on the spot and walking around for a few minutes.

2. Now, making sure you have a watch to time yourself, start walking your mile route at as brisk a pace as you can manage *without having to stop to get your breath back* and *still being able to talk*. (If you are on your own, count to ten now and then instead of talking!) You should feel your heart beating more strongly and should be aware of your lungs working harder to take in more air than normal. But you shouldn't feel any stress or pain in your chest or lungs, or any burning in your leg muscles.

If you do have to stop walking before the mile is up, that is the end of the test for today. You can try it again another day but at a slower pace so that you don't have to stop.

3. At the end of the mile, make a note of how long it took you to walk it. Check your results here:

Can't walk a mile: Very unfit indeed   ☐

Over 20 minutes: Unfit   ☐

18 – 20 minutes:	Quite unfit	☐
15 – 18 minutes:	Good level of fitness	☐
12 – 15 minutes:	Excellent level of fitness	☐
Under 12 minutes:	Superfit!	☐

The less fit you are, the more you will benefit from a gradual increase in your aerobic activity.

MUSCULAR STRENGTH AND TONE

The second corner of the fitness triangle is muscular strength. You have both small and large muscles all over your body, without which you wouldn't be able to move. If you *don't* take much exercise and they are under-used, they become smaller, stiffer and generally out of shape – and consequently, they make *you* look out of shape. People with poor muscle condition often think they need to lose weight when in fact they only need to tone up. If you're in good muscular condition, you will have a good overall appearance – sleek, firm and defined. Fit muscles also mean increased strength (so you can, for instance, carry heavier loads, or find that digging the garden is a less arduous task. But all this is relative – your basic body type, which is hereditary, will dictate how much muscular strength you can build up. Ectomorph types (basically skinny) can tone themselves up and look sleek and well proportioned but they are never going to be Schwarzenegger types. And if you are female you can do regular moderate muscular strength training without any fear of building up unsightly muscle.

To build up your muscle tone you need to do regular toning activity or a toning programme. Examples of muscle-toning activities include: the *Slim for Life* Flexi-Programme (see pages 248–282); swimming; gym workouts. And indeed all aerobic activity has some muscle-toning effect on some (but not all) parts of the body.

The benefits of muscular strength and tone

Now look through the list of benefits that increasing your muscular strength and tone can bring, and tick which ones you would particularly like to achieve:

☐ An increased proportion of lean body tissue (muscle) to fat means increased calorie burn-up and easier slimming. This is because muscle is more metabolically active than fat, so if you increase your muscle tissue your metabolic rate will be raised.

☐ Increased muscle tone makes your body look better – sleeker, slimmer and more in proportion – whatever your size. The main effects people notice are: a firmer, rounder bottom; a neater bustline; a smaller waist; a flatter stomach; firmer thighs; and firmer upper arms.

☐ Your posture will improve as toned muscles support your body in its correct position. Your shoulders will straighten and your stomach will pull in.

☐ Everyday aches and pains may lessen.

☐ Pelvic floor muscle exercises may help to cure stress incontinence.

☐ Your self-confidence will increase.

☐ Your ability to do everyday tasks will improve, e.g., carrying shopping, picking up children.

☐ You will gain increased protection against osteoporosis in older age.

Now try this strength and tone test. Wear clothes that don't restrict movement (e.g., leggings and T-shirt) and do the test in a warm room on a carpet, towel or mat.

MUSCULAR STRENGTH AND TONE TEST

1. Upper Body

- Kneel on all fours with your back straight and hands underneath shoulders, fingers pointing forwards.

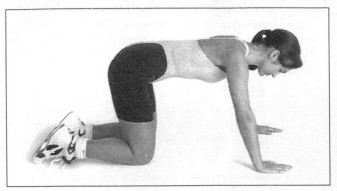

- Lower your chest towards the floor and rise up again, using the strength of your arms and chest.

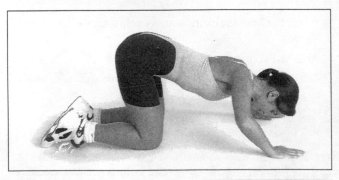

- How many of these push-ups can you do before muscle fatigue (weakness, shaking) sets in?

8 or more:	☐ Poor
9 – 20:	☐ Fair
Over 20:	☐ Good

2. *Stomach*

● Lie on your back with your knees bent and feet flat on the floor. Position your hands behind your head – supporting the neck but not grasping.

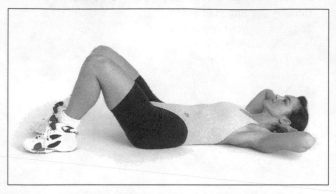

● Raise your head and shoulder blades off the floor.

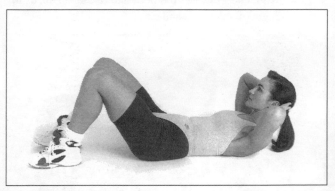

● Lower and repeat.
● How many of these crunches can you do before tiring?

8 or more: ☐	Poor
9 – 20: ☐	Fair
Over 20: ☐	Good

3. Legs

- Stand with feet hip distance apart, hands on your thighs.
- Lower your hips towards the floor by bending your knees and sticking your bottom out behind you. Stop when your legs are at a 45-degree angle to the floor.

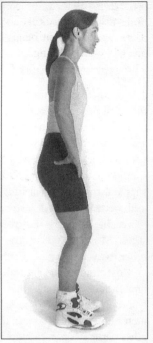

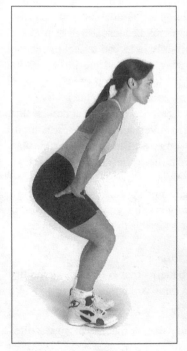

- Raise and repeat.
- How many of these squats can you do?

8 or more: ☐	Poor
9 – 20: ☐	Fair
Over 20: ☐	Good

The poorer your results in these tests, the more you will benefit from some simple strengthening and toning. The *Slim for Life* Flexi-Programme, beginning on page 248, is a graduated programme that can be done for as little as ten minutes three times a week, but other suggestions on how to increase your body strength and tone appear in the charts on pages 246–247.

FLEXIBILITY

The third corner of the fitness triangle is flexibility and is often the most neglected corner. Flexibility is your body's ability to move itself through a range of movement. Even people who are aerobically very fit with good body strength and tone can have very poor levels of flexibility. It is important to keep your spine, shoulders and hip joints flexible and mobile and your muscles supple throughout your life, not only because it will help you to look better but it will also certainly help you to feel better and more able to carry out everyday tasks and pastimes without strain. Muscles that are strengthened also need stretching out in order to avoid the risk of aches, pains and possible injury.

Most children are naturally flexible – it is only under-use that makes our bodies inflexible. However, some people are naturally more flexible than others. Women are often more flexible than men, and everyone has parts of the body that are less flexible than other parts. In order to increase your body's flexibility you need to do some regular stretching. Some sports and activities (e.g., yoga and dancing) will naturally involve you in stretching parts of your body. Most of us are less flexible than we may think.

The benefits of being flexible
Now look through the list of benefits that good body flexibility can bring you and tick which ones you would particularly like to achieve:

☐ Easing of minor aches and pains. Some may disappear altogether.

☐ Relaxation. If you're tense or nervous, a short aerobic workout or good warm-up followed by some stretches and deep breathing is a good way to relax.

Improved appearance. Stretching elongates tight and stiff muscles and can result in a sleeker overall appearance.

Ease of carrying out everyday activities (e.g., reaching and bending).

Avoidance of muscle stiffness. Stretching done after toning exercise prevents stiffness in the worked muscles the next day.

Improved posture. Many posture faults are due to short muscles that need to be worked (e.g., round shoulders due to short chest muscles; sway back due to tight hip flexors).

Improved enjoyment and performance at many pastimes, including dancing, tennis, and sex.

FLEXIBILITY TEST

Wear clothes that don't restrict movement and do the test in a warm room on a carpet, towel or mat. It is vital to be warm and relaxed before doing these tests.

1. Shoulders

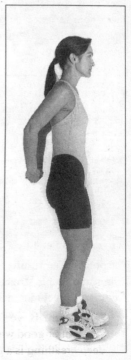

- Stand comfortably and clasp your fingers behind your back. Keeping your elbows bent, raise your arms still linked in this position.
- Use a mirror to judge your results.

Hands very close to
   your back: ☐ Poor
Hands 4 – 8 ins
   (10 – 20 cm) away: ☐ Fair
Hands over 8 ins
   (20 cm) away: ☐ Good

2. *Hamstrings and lower back*

- Sit with one leg straight out in front of you and the other leg bent and slightly to the side, foot on floor.

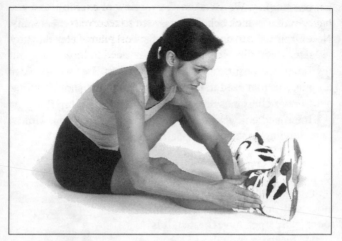

- Keeping your back straight (rather than curved forwards in a letter C-shape), lean over the straight leg as far as you can without pain. When you have leant as far as you can, reach your arms out and touch as far down the straight leg as you can. Don't hunch over with your shoulders to do this.

Around knee/calf level:	☐ Poor
Around ankle level:	☐ Fair
To sole of foot or beyond:	☐ Good

- How far can you reach?

The poorer your results in these tests, the more you will benefit from some simple stretching exercises. The *Slim for Life* Flexi-Programme includes a stretching section beginning on page 274, which should always be carried out after a few minutes' warm up (see page 252). Other suggestions for improving flexibility are included in the chart on pages 246–47.

The right choices for you

So now we are two-thirds of the way to finding out how best to get *you* moving. We've taken an overview of exercise, and you have decided which benefits *you* want to receive from activity. Now all we have to do is decide on the best plan of action to provide those benefits. To do this, first we need to look at all your own 'anti-exercise' prejudices (just as in Step Two we looked at all your excuses not to start a slimming campaign) and eliminate them or find ways round them.

These are the 'objections' I have encountered most often over the past ten years.

'I've no time to exercise'

Not being able to find time to fit exercise into a busy lifestyle is the single most frequent excuse I hear. If this sounds like you, first go back to Step Three (section 2) and read again why it is important to make time for yourself. Remember that you should consider it a priority every day to make mind time, food time and *body* time. Body time is the time when you could take activity – if not every day, then at least three times a week. If you're still not managing daily 'body time' – then *try* ... and keep trying. Once you get into the habit of 'time for you' it's easier, especially if you plan ahead. Each morning as soon as you wake up decide what you're going to do for your body, and when, and stick to it.

Also bear in mind that many people who start to take regular exercise report that as a result they actually accomplish more in a day than they did before. The exercise refreshes them and 'sharpens them up', so they achieve more – thus *saving* time!

Next, when time is at a premium, consider your exercise priorities. Depending on your results in the fitness assessments earlier in this Step, it may be that you need more work on one aspect of the 'fitness triangle' than another. If your flexibility is poor but your aerobic fitness is good, then concentrate on improving your flexibility.

You can also use the Activity Chart on pages 246–247 to pick activities that exercise each part of the fitness triangle to some degree. For example, dancing is good for aerobic fitness, strength and tone *and* suppleness, so this would save your having to do two or more different types of exercise to improve or maintain overall fitness. Cycling, on the other hand, is good for aerobic fitness and leg strength but will not improve upper body strength or flexibility, so you would have to combine cycling with flexibility and upper body exercises, taking up more of your time.

If your time is genuinely short, don't be pushed into the trap of thinking that to be fit you *need* to spend ages on a programme – you don't. Just one hour a week divided, say, into three ten-minute toning and stretch sessions (as in the Flexi-Programme starting on page 248), plus three ten-minute aerobic sessions (e.g., brisk walking) will make you fitter if your current fitness level is very poor. More time might be better – but doing *something* is always better than doing *nothing* when time is limited. Also remember you can do more exercise in your less busy weeks, and do a 'hold' programme on very busy weeks.

Lastly, reconsider your attitude to 'exercise'. To get fitter, it's not necessary to do a set, regular, formal programme or class. You can get much fitter – and burn up many extra calories – by simply building more activity into your daily life. Run up the stairs instead of walking (saving time here too!); practise contracting and releasing the muscles in your bottom when sitting at a desk or table, or do ankle-circling for improved joint mobility. Get into the habit of being more aware of your body throughout the day and moving it whenever you get the chance. If you're standing waiting for something or someone, do some semi-squats or practise a pelvic tilt – pulling your tummy and bottom in to correct an over-concave lower back. If you're in the kitchen waiting for the kettle to boil, do some heel-raises to firm up your calves, or clasp your hands behind your back and pull your arms back for an easy chest stretch exercise. Your body is waiting to be used – use it *anytime*, not just at formal exercise sessions! (However, always try to make sure your body is warm if you're doing spur-of-the-moment exercises to avoid any chance of strains.)

'Exercise is boring'

This is the second most common reason people cite for not exercising! I used to think exercise was boring until I saw how much nicer my body looked and how much better it felt when I *did* exercise. The simple truth is that whatever activities you do, you've *got* to pick ones you enjoy.

There is so much choice available that I am never quite sure why people do embark on exercise classes or routines or sports that they don't like. Use the Activity Chart on pages 246–247 to select a form of exercise you enjoy. And, remember, you don't always have to stick with the same choice – vary your activities to prevent boredom setting in. For aerobic fitness, you can combine walking with cycling and swimming or stepping. In fact there is an extra benefit to doing this, since you will also be using slightly different muscles for the various aerobic activities, thus achieving a better all-round toning and strengthening effect.

Another way to prevent boredom setting in is to pick those activities you can do with other people. For instance, you could join a walking or cycling club (or even form your own), go to an exercise class with a friend, or (when you are reasonably fit) take up competition in your chosen sport. Really, the only limit to the possibilities is your own mind!

Lastly, people with a low boredom threshold will find my earlier advice on building more activity into your daily life very useful. If you have a mental block about 'formal' exercise, the idea that you can improve your fitness while you go about your everyday life is an appealing one.

There's no need to be a slave to exercise, so make sure you set yourself reasonable exercise targets, say, three short sessions a week of something you like, rather than impossible ones you'll never stick to, such as an hour a day doing a floor routine to a video. Remember, it's much better to do a little of something you like, than a lot of something you don't like – and then give up!

'Exercise is too hard for me'

If on previous occasions you've tried exercise and found it too difficult, or it resulted in too many aches and pains afterwards, then the answer is simple: you were doing exercise that wasn't at a suitable level for your ability, or the exercise was a type I wouldn't recommend.

Unless you have a particular illness or disability that prevents you from exercising (and if you think you have, or if you have any doubts, you should see your doctor for a check-up and get his or her okay first), there is no reason why you cannot start an exercise programme. The simplest aerobic activity is usually walking. Anyone can do this, however unfit they may be. You simply walk for a short distance to begin with, at a pace that gets your heart and lungs working a little but that allows you to carry on a conversation. No matter if everyone else can walk faster or for longer – and you shouldn't compete against anyone if you are not fit – just aim gradually to improve your own fitness.

All the latest research shows that for most people, *moderate* activity is just as good as, if not better than, *vigorous* activity. Swimming is another good option if you are not fit. And the *Slim for Life* Flexi-Programme on page 248 offers a good tone and stretch workout suitable for beginners.

Remember, if you end up with aching muscles and feeling tired and terrible after exercise then you've done too much. Most people I know who complain of this feeling have simply done something very active after a long period of inaction e.g., a day's digging after six months of doing nothing; a morning's playing cricket after a ten-year absence from the game, or a sponsored five-mile walk when a hundred yards down to the shop is as far as you usually go!

You've got to be sensible about starting activity when you are unfit. *Easy* does it; *gradual* does it and *never mind* if you can't do much to start with – honestly, you will soon improve. And that applies to older people just as much as to young ones.

'I'm too embarrassed to exercise'

If people are out of condition, or overweight, or both, they are often worried about being 'shown up' at an exercise class full of 'slim fitties', or being stared at as they make a feeble attempt at swimming for the first time in years.

Well, I can understand that. If you refuse to exercise through inhibitions of this kind, the obvious thing to do is pick an activity that you can do in privacy at home – at least to start with. A floor routine such as the Slim for Life Flexi-Programme beginning on page 248 will get you toned and more supple. Combine that with a regular walk (or, if you can afford it, buy a step to use at home plus a stepping video for routine ideas) and you can get fit with no embarrassment at all! Later on you may like to try other activities. And don't forget, if you do venture to the pool or to an exercise class, other people are usually more interested in their own performance than in looking at anyone else. If it helps, take a friend along for moral support, and make sure you choose a beginners' class where everyone is likely to be at a similar level to you.

If you are overweight, there is no reason why you should not exercise, unless your doctor says otherwise. It will help your weight-loss campaign and help you to avoid the 'flabby bits' that people who slim without exercise often get left with.

'I can't afford to exercise'

Activity doesn't have to be expensive – it can be free. A regular programme of walking plus the strength/tone and stretch exercises on pages 260–282 will cost you nothing. Skipping is inexpensive and so is cycling if you already have a bike. There are many sports and exercise classes which are relatively inexpensive, such as local authority classes and sports facilities like badminton, netball, swimming and tennis. Some exercise will even save you money. Why not try cycling to work instead of taking a bus or train; or walking to the shops instead of using the car?

Of course, there are always expensive activities – exclusive gyms with high membership fees, golf clubs, skiing and horse-riding. If you have limited finances, pick an activity that is low-cost but please don't use money as a reason *not* to exercise!

'I'm stuck with pre-school children every day – I can't possibly exercise'

Well you *can* – you just have to be a bit more resourceful about what you choose and when you do it. Pushing a push-chair or pram is a good way of exercising. Many mums I know do an indoor floor routine (like the Flexi-Programme beginning on page 248) when their babies and toddlers are having an afternoon nap or after they've gone to bed at night. Some local authority leisure centres provide crèche facilities. And there are many mother and baby or toddler swim sessions.

And, if you have a partner, is there no time (e.g., at weekends) when that partner could take over with some child-minding so that you could get out and do your roller-skating or horse-riding, or whatever it is that you would really like to do but can't take the children with you?

Go through the Activity Chart on pages 246–247 and consider what activities you can do – and stop worrying about the ones you can't until the children are older. Meanwhile, enjoy taking them to the park and playing catch, rounders or chase. You can get fit that way, too!

'I don't see any results when I exercise so there is no incentive'

Perhaps you have been doing activity that is too easy for your ability. Just as an unfit person needs to start gently and gradually work up, you will also need to increase the level of difficulty of your fitness activity once you reach a certain level. Exercise is not aerobic unless you are increasing your heart rate and your oxygen intake while you do it. Therefore, if a walk on the level at, say, 4 mph (6.4 kph) doesn't have that effect, then it won't improve your fitness, and you will need to walk for longer or faster, walk uphill or walk with weights, until you reach a level that is aerobic.

Similarly, if you can lift a set of 22 lb (10 kg) weights repeatedly with ease, that weight isn't going to improve your strength at all. You need to increase the weight to see further improvement.

Once you've reached a certain level of fitness, you need to *increase* the number of sessions a week or spend more *time* exercising, or work *harder* to achieve better results.

Now all you have to do is look through the Activity Chart that follows and decide on an initial 'course of action'.

Using the Activity Chart

Using the discussions on the last few pages, together with the results of your fitness assessment, make a note of your basic, most important requirements of a fitness programme. For example, you may decide 'low cost/high aerobic benefit/something I can do in private/in a few spare minutes at odd times of the day.

Look down the chart and you'll see the following activities would fit in well with those requirements: stair climbing/skipping/aerobic video routine (e.g, aerobic section of the *Y-Plan*). For a little more money you could also consider a rebounder (mini-trampoline) or a step.

Someone else may have different priorities (e.g., all-round fitness regime I can do in twenty minutes a day, with variety in it so I don't get bored/not too difficult). For that person I would suggest three aerobic sessions a week – two walking, one swimming or cycling, plus three tone and stretch sessions. The *Slim for Life* Flexi-Programme would be ideal for at least two of those sessions, and, if a swim was included, that would count as a tone and stretch session as well. The last day would be a rest day.

Your requirements

....

....

....

....

How much time?

The absolute minimum I would suggest for a fitness improvement in a fairly unfit person is approximately one hour a week of 'structured' exercise, plus as much 'building extra activity into your daily routine' as you can (see pages 237–239 for more ideas).

Unless the fitness tests showed you to be 'unevenly' fit (i.e., fit in two corners of the triangle but not in the third), you should split that hour of structured exercise into half an hour of aerobic activity and half an hour of strength/tone and stretch activity. And you should split each of those half hours up as evenly throughout the week as you can (e.g., three ten-minute sessions of strength/tone and stretch and two fifteen-minute or three ten-minute sessions of aerobics.

Even with just one hour's exercise a week, as long as you keep trying to improve (i.e., in the case of aerobic activity, going further or more quickly, or in the case of strength/tone and stretch, doing the harder exercises or doing the movements better) you will see a gradual build-up of all-round fitness.

But obviously if you can find more time, then so much the better. The majority of fitness experts agree that three twenty-minute aerobic sessions a week are ideal to improve aerobic fitness. So if you can find ninety minutes a week, you could do three twenty-minute aerobic sessions and three ten-minute strength/tone and stretch sessions, or three aerobic sessions and one thirty-minute strength/tone and stretch class, perhaps. You work out a programme that suits *you* – and remember, you don't have to do exactly the same every week.

However, if you feel you really would like me to tell you exactly what to do, then this is what I would recommend: walking is the ideal aerobic activity for most people (ten minutes three times a week, building up to thirty minutes three times a week); and the *Slim for Life* Flexi-Programme is sufficient for most people to improve strength/tone and suppleness (ten minutes a day three times a week, building up to twenty minutes three times a week). But I would rather *you* made the choice – and you *can* take control of your own activity programme, I promise you!

Meaning of symbols on the chart
The Activity Chart enables you to see at a glance what fitness benefits you will get from any activity.

Each activity is rated for its ability to improve your fitness in all the corners of the triangle – aerobic, upper body strength and tone; lower body strength and tone; and flexibility:

>   * Little or no effect
>   ** A reasonably good effect
>   *** An excellent effect

For all-round fitness you should try to do activities each week that have a good or excellent effect on each of the fitness corners. For instance, if you were to choose only cycling, your aerobic fitness would improve and so would your lower body strength, but you'd be doing little for your upper body or overall flexibility. Therefore you would need to choose extra activities to raise your star level in those particular corners. And if you were to choose the *Slim for Life* Flexi-Programme, you would also need to pick some aerobic activity to complement it, as it has little or no effect on your aerobic fitness.

In addition, the chart tells you roughly how many calories per minute you will burn for that activity, and in the last column it gives a suitability rating for your level of fitness:

    * Suitable for people who aren't very fit/beginners
   ** Suitable for people who are reasonably fit
*** Don't take up this activity until you are fit

This chart is intended as a guide only and you should use your common sense to pick an activity that suits your ability. (e.g., an aerobics class may be fine for a beginner, providing it is billed as a 'beginners' class').

Activity Chart

Activity	Aerobic	Strength/tone upper body	Strength/tone lower body	Flexibility	Calories per minute	Rating
Aerobics class	***	**	***	**	7	**
Archery	*	**	*	*	3	*
Badminton	**	**	**	*	5	*
Basketball	**	**	**	*	5	**
Body conditioning class	**	***	***	***	4	*
Circuit training (in gym)	***	***	***	**	5	**
Cricket	*	**	**	*	3	**
Cycling	***	*	***	*	7	**
Dancing (slow)	**	*	**	**	4	*
Dancing (disco or Latin type)	***	**	**	**	5	*
Digging	*	**	**	*	4	**
Fencing	**	**	**	*	5	**
Football	**	*	**	*	5	**
Golf	**	**	**	*	4	*
Gymnastics	**	***	***	***	5	**
Handball	**	**	**	*	4	*
Hockey	**	**	**	*	5	**
Horse riding	*	**	***	*	4	*
Housework	*	**	**	**	4	*

Activity	Aerobic	Strength/tone upper body	Strength/tone lower body	Flexibility	Calories per minute	Rating
Ice skating	**	*	***	**	4	**
Jogging	***	*	***	*	7	***
Judo	*	**	**	***	4	**
Mowing grass (push along powered mower)	***	**	**	*	5	*
Rock climbing	***	*	***	**	4	**
Roller skating	***	*	***	*	5	**
Rowing	***	***	**	*	7	***
Rugby	**	**	**	*	6	**
Running	***	*	***	*	8	***
Skiing (cross country)	***	***	***	*	8	***
Skiing (downhill)	**	**	***	*	6	**
Skipping (rope)	***	**	***	*	6	*
Slim for Life Flexi-Programme	*	***	***	***	3	*
Squash	**	**	***	*	10	***
Stair climbing or stepping	***	*	***	*	8	**
Stretch classes	*	*	*	***	3	**
Swimming	***	***	***	**	7	**
Table tennis	**	**	**	*	5	*
Tennis	**	**	***	*	6	**
Volleyball	**	**	**	*	5	*
Walking	***	*	***	*	5	*
Weight lifting	*	***	**	*	7	***
Yoga	*	*	*	***	3	**
Yomping (alternating walk with jog)	***	*	***	*	6	**

Note: Performing stretches following most of the above activities is a sensible precaution against injury and will also mean that particular activity gives you flexibility benefits.

The Slim for Life Flexi-Programme

The strength/tone and stretch Flexi-Programme that follows is the simplest-ever way to get – or maintain – basic body strength, tone and suppleness.

It is totally flexible in terms of fitness ability and available time. You can begin it, however unfit you are, with no fear of over-taxing your ability, and you can follow this programme whether you have ten minutes a few times a week to spare, or much more (up to thirty minutes six times a week).

If you combine it with one of the aerobic activities listed on pages 246–247 (walking is simple and ideal), you can become totally fit *in your own time*.

The Flexi-Programme has other advantages too – it costs nothing and can be done almost anywhere. Here's how it works:

THE WARM-UP

Like every good body-conditioning routine, the Flexi-Programme begins with a warm-up. Everyone should do this – it takes only a few minutes – and is vital for warming the large muscle groups to prepare them for the movements ahead and to prevent possible injury. It should also raise your heartbeat slightly and leave you literally feeling warm.

THE ROUTINE

Next there is the 'core' toning routine. This consists of only six different exercises which, between them, work all the major muscle groups of your body. You don't *need* to do lots of different exercises for each part of the body, so I've cut this routine right down to the basics to make it easy to follow and simple to do.

Each of the six exercises has three different levels of ability. Level One is the easiest, and everyone should begin on this level. Level Two is a slightly harder version of the basic Level One move and should be attempted when the Level One move becomes easy. Level Three is harder still and should be attempted when you have mastered the Level Two move.

THE COOL-DOWN STRETCHES

The last part of the programme contains a set of gentle stretches, which also act as a cool-down, leaving you feeling refreshed and relaxed. Since your body will be well warmed up after the core exercise routine you will find it easier to stretch it into the movements.

There are nine stretches covering all parts of the body, and doing them for a few minutes at the end of the routine will ensure that you have no aches and pains the next day, as well as increasing your body's flexibility.

HOW MUCH TIME SHOULD YOU SPEND ON THE FLEXI-PROGRAMME?

The complete routine (including warm-up and stretches) should take a minimum of ten minutes. This is based on three minutes each for the warm-up and cool-down stretches, and four minutes to complete *one set* of each of the six core exercises. *One set* means each exercise is repeated *eight times* in a slow and controlled manner.

I suggest that everyone starts with this ten-minute, one-set routine, at least for the first week or two. After that, you can simply stick with ten minutes per session, gradually increasing the difficulty of the programme as you get fitter by moving through Levels Two and Three, and by improving the positions in which you hold the cool-down stretches.

Alternatively, you can increase the number of sets you do of the core exercises. To do this you repeat an exercise eight times for one set, then stop and take a rest for ten to fifteen seconds before doing another set of eight. Doing the whole routine with *two sets* will take you approximately fifteen minutes, with *three* sets, about twenty minutes, and so on. You can do as many sets as you like as long as you build up gradually and don't attempt too much too soon.

Obviously, the more sets you do and the sooner you move through the levels to the harder exercises, the quicker you will build muscle strength and tone.

HOW OFTEN SHOULD YOU DO THE ROUTINE?

The minimum I recommend for acceptable results is three times a week of the basic ten-minute routine. That amounts to just half an hour a week! However, if you choose to do the routine more often than that, again, you will become fitter more quickly. You can do it up to six times a week if you wish, but initially I suggest you start with three times a week of the basic ten-minute routine and see how you go.

Eventually, you can build up to thirty minutes six times a week, if you like, or you can simply do the ten-minute routine three times a week indefinitely for basic strength and tone maintenance. It may be that some weeks you do more, other weeks less. Always remember that a little activity done regularly is much, much better than doing none at all.

To sum up these are the ways you can tailor the Flexi-Programme to suit your needs:

1. There are three levels of ability for each of the six core exercises (Level One, easy; Level Two, harder; Level Three, hardest). You do the one that suits your current fitness level and move to the next one as you improve.
2. You do from one to five sets of each exercise depending on how much time you have. One set is eight repetitions, and the ten-minute routine contains one set of each core exercise. Five sets will increase the total time for the whole routine to thirty minutes.

3. You decide how many times a week you do the routine. A ten-minute routine three times a week performed regularly will achieve results.

TIPS TO HELP YOU

- Exercise in a warm room and wear comfortable, non-restrictive clothing.
- Make sure the floor is not too hard and, if it is not carpeted, use a good, thick, non-slip mat to exercise on.
- Don't exercise if you are ill.
- Breathe comfortably throughout.
- Concentrate as you do the movements; do them in a slow and controlled way.
- Move into a stretch and hold the position, rather than doing repeated bounces.
- If you are doing the programme properly – and moving up through the levels when you are ready – the routine should make you feel that your body is working, but there should be no pain. If you reach a stage during the core routine when the muscle you are exercising begins to shake, then stop – you have done enough.
- When doing the stretches, you should feel a pleasant, warm sensation in the muscle(s) being stretched, but not a nasty burning. It is important to try to breathe deeply and relax into the stretch. You may then be able to achieve a bigger stretch without strain. Stop if any muscle hurts.

Do not begin this programme until you have read the preceding pages and understand what you should be doing.

The Flexi warm-up

Starting Position
- Stand with your
feet slightly apart,
knees relaxed and
pointing in the
same direction as
your toes. Keep
your back straight,
stomach pulled in
and shoulders back
and down.

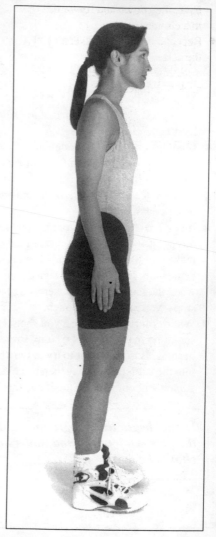

1. *Shoulder rolls*

- Lift the shoulders up and back, then down and forwards in a circular motion.
- Repeat 8 times, then reverse the action in a forwards direction 8 times. Feel the neck and upper back loosen up.

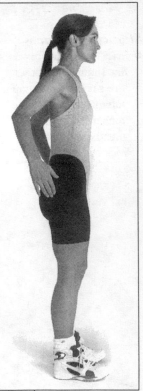

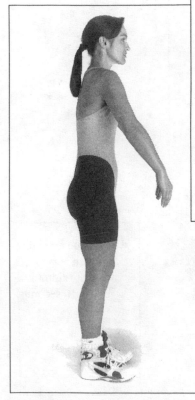

2. Marching

● March on the spot,
  pumping your arms
  backwards and forwards
  for 1 minute. Start with
  low marches and gradually
  raise knees higher and
  higher until you are
  breathing deeply.

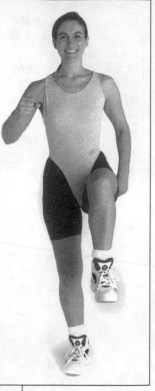

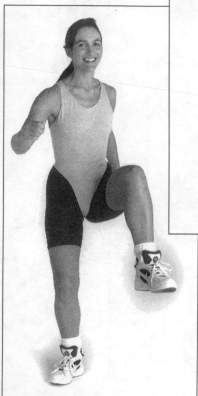

● Continue marching
  but with legs in a
  wide position for a
  further 10 seconds.

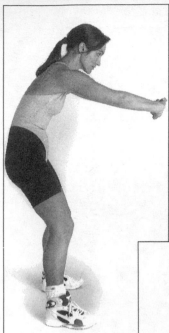

3. *Low-back release*
- Keep the feet in the wide position, extend your arms forwards at shoulder level and link hands loosely. Everything else is in the starting position.
- Let the knees bend a little further as you curl the back into a letter C-shape and pull the stomach in. Hold for 10 seconds. Release and repeat.

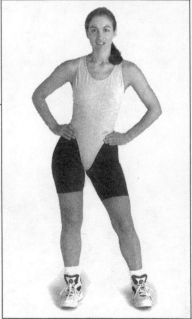

4. *Hip circles*
- In the starting position, but with feet wide, imagine you have a hula hoop and circle your hips very slowly a few times, first in a clockwise direction and then in an anti-clockwise direction.

5. *Side to side sway and reach for the sky*

- With the feet still in the wide position shift your weight from side to side, bending the knee of the leg you are moving as you come up on the toes of the opposite foot. As you move to the right, lift your left arm up and across, palm facing forwards, changing arms as you sway to the other side.
- Repeat 20 times, 10 to each side alternately.

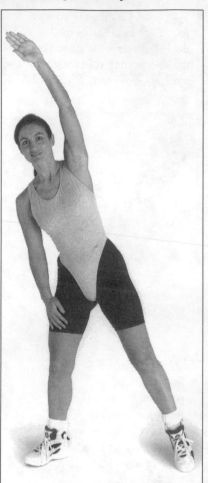

6. Step touch with arm swings

- Take your weight on to your left foot and bring your right foot in to touch beside it. As you do so, swing your arms to the left. Reverse the movement by taking your right foot to the side, putting your weight on it and bringing the left foot in to touch beside it. Swing the arms across at the same time.

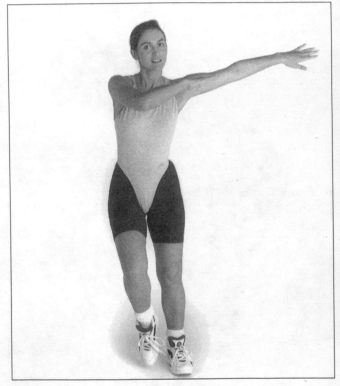

- Repeat 20 times in all, 10 to each side with the arms flowing from side to side. You can clap if you like as the arms swing to the side.

7. *Hamstring and calf stretch*

- Bend your left knee and take your right leg out in front of you. Keeping your right leg straight, lean over it, bending from the hips and supporting your body with your hands on your left thigh. Feel the stretch in the back of the right thigh. Lift your right toes to add a mid-calf stretch. Hold for 10 seconds.
- Repeat with the other leg in front.

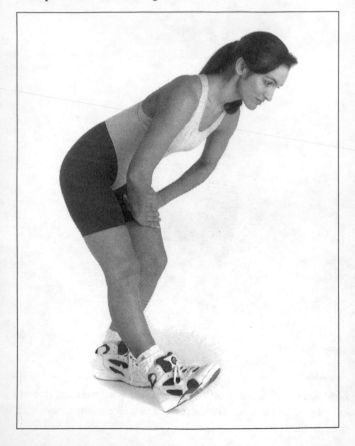

8. *Quadricep stretch*

- Stand in the starting position and hold on to a chair or stool with your left hand (or place your left hand against a wall to support yourself). Grasp the middle part of your right foot (or your right heel) with your right hand and bring it towards your bottom. Feel the front of your thigh stretch out. Hold for 8 seconds.
- Repeat with the other leg.

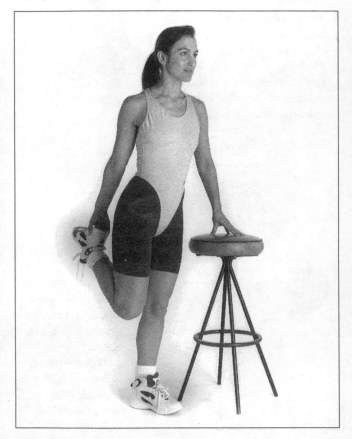

Strength and Tone

Now you are warmed up you can begin the strength and tone exercises. Remember, if you are new to this routine, start on Level One for each of the six exercises.

1. SQUATS: FOR THIGHS AND BOTTOM

Level One
- Stand in the starting position.
- Bend your knees until your thighs are approximately at a 45-degree angle to the floor, reaching your arms forwards to aid balance. Your back should remain straight, although at a diagonal angle since your hips will stick out behind you.

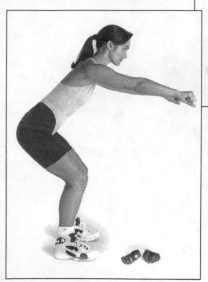

- Slowly return to the starting position and repeat 8 times. (If you can't go down that far to begin with, just go as far as you can until you feel your thigh and bottom muscles working.)

Level Two
- As Level One but this time squatting down further until your thighs are almost parallel to the floor, if possible. Do not go any lower than this point.
- Repeat 8 times slowly for one set.

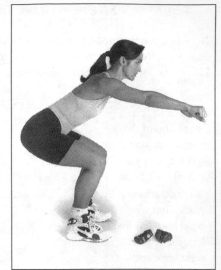

Level Three
- As Level Two but adding some arm strengthening work. Pick up your handweights (or cans of beans). Keep your elbows by your sides and bring your hands towards your shoulders as you squat down. Return hands to your sides as you raise up.
- Repeat 8 times slowly for one set.

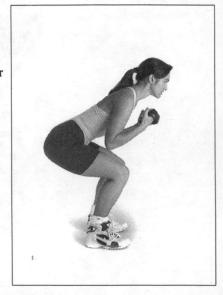

2. LEG SWEEPS: FOR OUTER THIGHS, HIPS AND BOTTOM

Level One

- Stand side on to a sturdy chair or stool. Hold the back of the chair or the top of the stool with your left hand (or use a wall for support) and place your right hand on your hip. Place your right leg a few inches in front of you, pointing the toes so the toes just touch the floor.

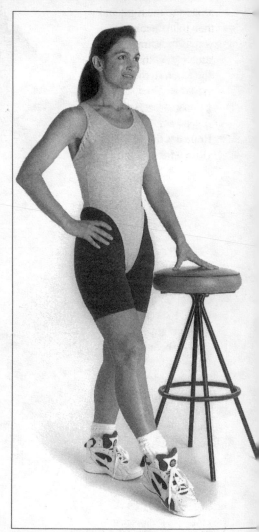

- In a sweeping motion, bring your right leg around to the right and then to the back of you, all the time keeping the toes in contact with the floor to aid balance. Reverse the movement to sweep the leg around to the front again, and repeat 8 times.

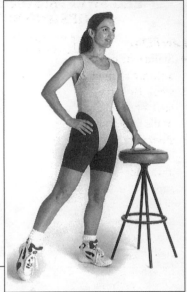

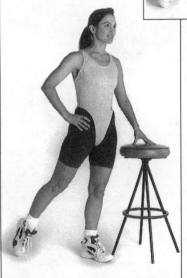

- Turn around and repeat 8 times with your left leg for a complete set.

Level Two

- Use an exercise rubber band or a tied Dyna-Band. Place the band around your ankles. Perform the exercise 8 times with each leg, sweeping the leg around as before.

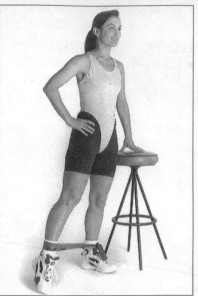

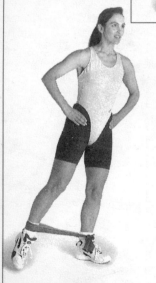

Level Three

- As Level Two but without support. Keep your body stabilized by holding your stomach back and bottom muscles tight as you perform the exercise. (You can also tie the Dyna-Band into a shorter circle or use a stronger rubber band to make the exercise harder.) Perform the exercise 8 times with each leg.

3. CRUNCHES: FOR THE STOMACH (ABDOMINALS)

Level One (Basic crunch)

- Lie on your back with your knees bent, feet flat on the floor. Rest your hands on your thighs, or have them behind the base of your head. (This latter arm position makes the crunch a little more difficult but helps support the weight of the head and may prevent neck ache.)

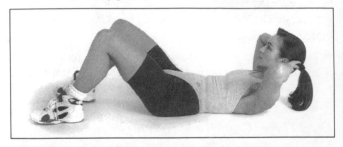

- Slowly raise the head and shoulder blades off the floor, using the abdominal muscles to make a curling action and bringing the rib cage towards the thighs.
- Lower, and repeat 8 times for one set.

Level Two (Reverse curl)

- Lie flat, bring your knees into the chest with ankles crossed and feet relaxed down towards the thighs. Have your hands behind your head.

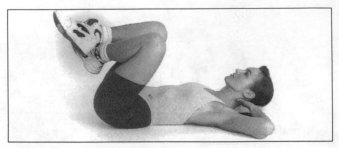

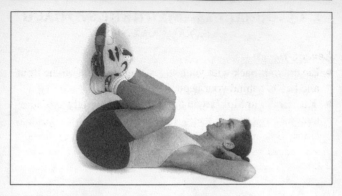

- Pull in the abdominal muscles so that the hips move towards your rib cage – it is a rolling action rather than a pushing-up action. Be careful not to swing the legs.
- Repeat 8 times for one set.

Level Three (Crunch and reverse curl)
- Start in the same position as Level Two.
- Combine the movements of Levels One and Two by lifting your head and shoulders off the floor, bringing your rib cage towards your knees as you also use the abdominal muscles to roll the hips in.

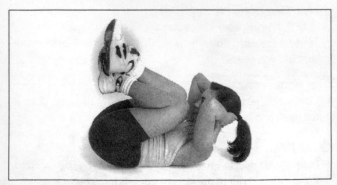

- Repeat 8 times for one set.

4. DIAGONAL CURLS: FOR THE STOMACH (ABDOMINALS)

Level One

- Lie on your back with your knees bent, feet flat on the floor and hands behind your head.
- Keeping your hips flat on the floor, take the right shoulder over towards the left knee – you can lead with the right elbow. The other elbow should be on the floor to give you support as you lift. Lower, and reverse sides.

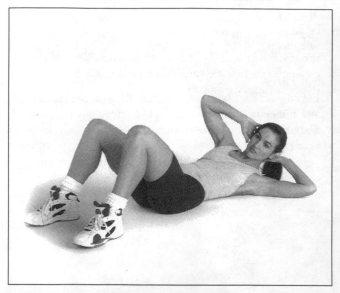

- Continue repeating to each side alternately, 16 times in total for one set.

Level Two

- Lie on your back with the soles of your feet together and knees relaxed out to the sides, your left hand behind your head.

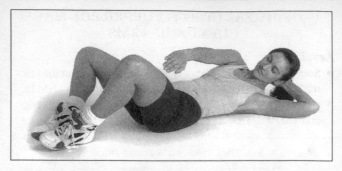

- Reach the right arm towards the right knee, aiming the right shoulder towards the left thigh. Lower, and reverse sides.
- Repeat to each side alternately, 16 times in total for one set.

Level Three

- Lie on your back with your legs raised in the air, knees bent and ankles crossed, ensuring that your legs stay above the body and do not extend beyond it. Place your hands behind your head.

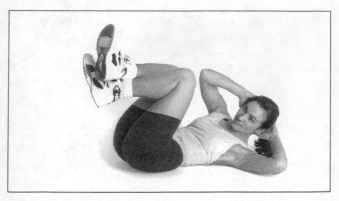

- Take the right shoulder across towards the outside of the left thigh, leading with both elbows. Lower, and reverse sides.
- Repeat to each side alternately, 16 times in total for one set.

5. PRESS-UPS: FOR UPPER BODY, CHEST AND ARMS

Level One

● Start by kneeling on all fours with thighs at right angles to the floor. Your back is straight and your stomach pulled in. Ensure that your wrists are in line with your shoulders and that your fingers are pointing forwards.

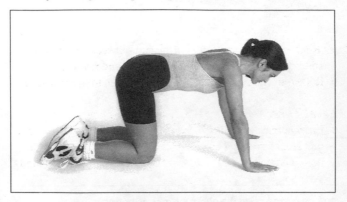

● Lower the chest towards the floor. Go as far as you can, then slowly return to the starting position.

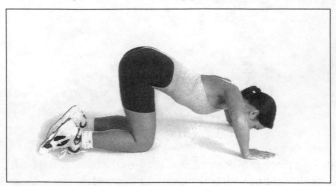

● Repeat 8 times for one set.

Level Two

● Kneel as before but with your hands and shoulders further forwards and your ankles lifted so that your bottom is halfway to the floor.

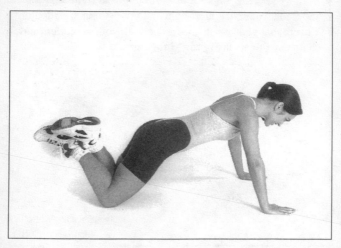

● Lower and raise the chest 8 times as before.

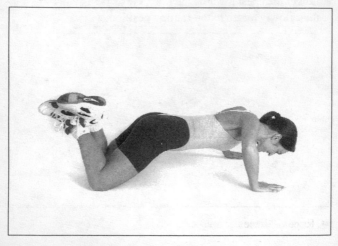

Level Three

- Start with your legs straight, hips slightly lifted and wrists in line with your shoulders.

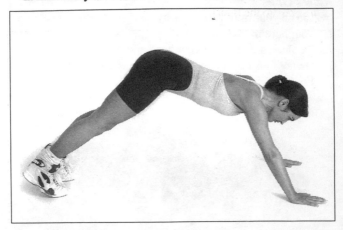

- Slowly lower your chest to the floor, then raise up. Keep your back straight, hips slightly lifted and stomach in. This is a full press-up.

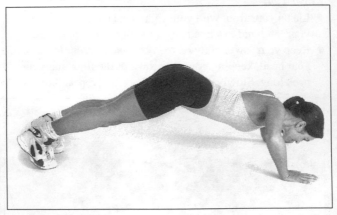

- Repeat 8 times.

6. BACK EXTENSIONS: FOR THE LOWER BACK

Level One
- Lie on your front with arms by your sides, hands resting on your bottom. Keeping your hips and legs firmly anchored to the floor, slowly raise your head and shoulders off the floor. Do not look up, but keep your face towards the floor. Lower, and repeat.

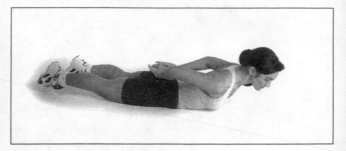

- Repeat 8 times for one set.

Level Two
- Lie on your front with your right hand under your head and your left hand extended along the floor in front of you.
- Keep your lower body on the floor and lift your left arm and your head, keeping your face towards the floor and your neck long. Slowly return to the floor, and repeat 8 times.

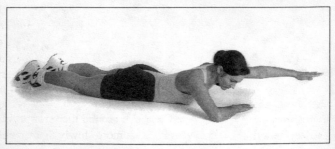

- Change sides and perform the exercise 8 times, lifting the right arm.

Level Three
- As Level Two, but as the left arm lifts, raise the right leg, still ensuring the hips stay in contact with the floor. Slowly return to the floor, and repeat 8 times.

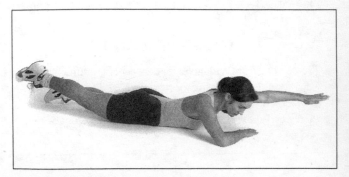

- Change sides, and repeat 8 times. (This exercise also strengthens the muscles of the bottom.)

Stretch and Cool-Down

Hold each of the following stretches for a minimum of 10 seconds. As you get used to the stretches you can stay in them for 30 seconds each. As you become more supple you will be able to develop a better stretch. The photos are only a guide, so don't worry if you cannot reach as far to start with – muscles that have not been worked for a while take time to develop flexibility.

1. ABDOMINAL STRETCH

- Lie on your front and have your arms bent, palms beside your shoulders. Keeping the neck long and forearms in contact with the floor, raise the chest and shoulders. Hold, then slowly lower. Feel this stretch along the front of your body.

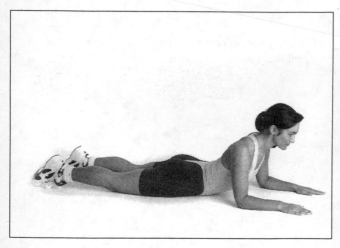

2. FRONT THIGH (QUADRICEP) STRETCH

- Lying on your front, hold the middle of your right foot or its heel with your right hand and bring it in towards your hips. Make sure you keep the knees together and your hips in contact with the floor. (If, initially, you are not able to reach your foot, wrap a towel around the foot and hold both ends to bring the foot in towards the body.) Hold, then release.

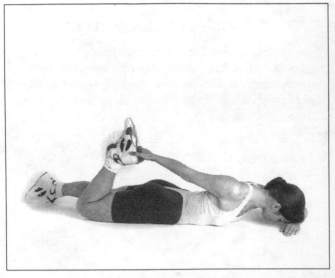

- Repeat with the other foot. You will feel this stretch along the front of your thigh.

3. BACK STRETCH SEQUENCE

This sequence will give you a pleasant stretch all along the back.

- Start on all fours with hands under your shoulders, and arch your back like a cat. Hold, then slowly return to a flat back.

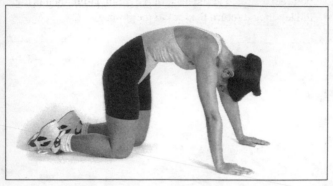

- From all fours, slowly lower the hips down on to the calves, then lower the chest to the floor as you slide the hands forwards. Hold.

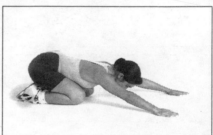

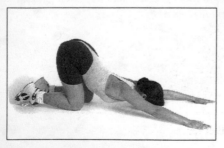

- To increase this stretch, raise the hips off the calves. You may also be able to slide the fingers further forwards.

4. BACK OF THIGH (HAMSTRING) STRETCH

- Lie on your back with both knees bent and feet flat on the floor.
- With one hand on your left calf, bring the left knee in towards your chest, then slowly straighten the left leg until you feel a stretch at the back of the thigh. Hold, then bring the leg in and return the foot to the floor.

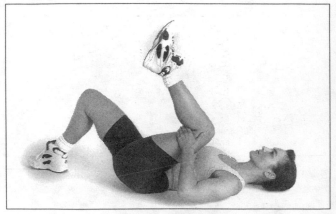

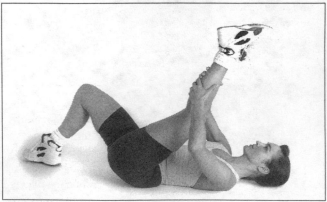

- Repeat with the other leg.

5. INNER THIGH STRETCH

● Sitting up (on a mat or a towel if this is more comfortable), place the soles of the feet together and let the knees fall to the sides. Hold loosely on to the calves or feet and let your elbows press gently on to your knees, easing them towards the floor. You will feel the stretch along the inner thighs. As you progress, your knees will come nearer to the floor.

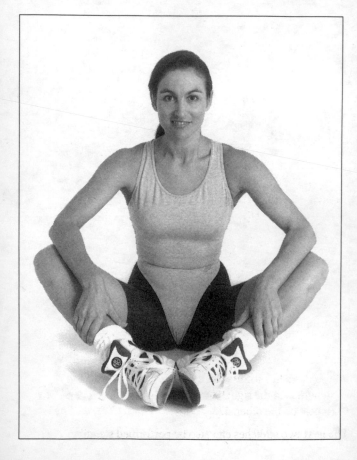

6. OUTER THIGH AND HIP STRETCH

- Sit with your left leg extended in front of you, bend the right leg and cross it over the left. Hold your right leg with your left arm and gently ease the knee into your body. You will feel a stretch along the right hip and outer thigh.

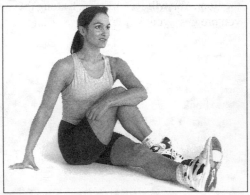

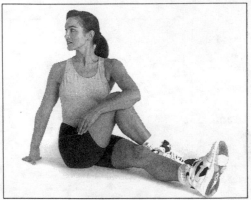

- You can add a torso stretch by turning your head and shoulders to the right. Hold, then slowly uncurl.
- Repeat on the other side.

The next two stretches can also be performed standing.

7. CHEST STRETCH

- Sit with your legs in a comfortable position for you and your back straight. Link hands behind your back and, keeping your elbows bent, slowly extend the arms behind you, pulling the shoulder blades together. You will feel this stretch through your chest.

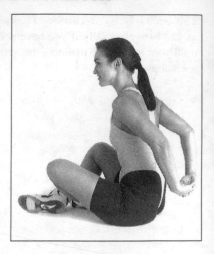

8. TRICEP STRETCH

- Still sitting comfortably, bend your left arm, trying to keep the elbow close to your head. Apply gentle pressure to the arm to increase the stretch. Hold.
- Repeat on the other side.

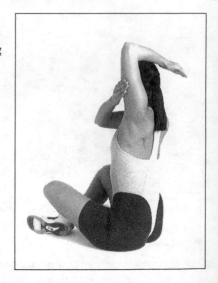

9. LONG BODY STRETCH

This stretch is my favourite and feels great. Hold it for as long as you can, especially if you have poor posture as it will help train your muscles to maintain their correct positions when you are standing.

- Lie on your back with your knees bent and your arms outstretched on the floor above your head. If you have a tight chest or tight shoulders you will find it impossible to get your arms and your back on the floor. If that is the case, carefully raise your back off the floor so that you can get your arms on the floor, then slowly press your back into the floor again, concentrating on keeping your arms flat for as long as possible. Over the weeks you will gradually be able to stretch out flat from your bottom up to your fingertips. As you stretch, you will feel your stomach really flattening towards your spine and your chest expanding.

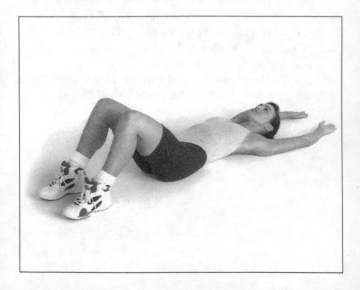

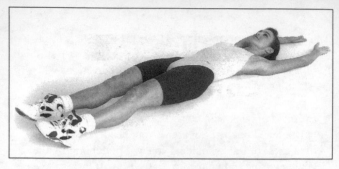

- After holding this position for a minimum of 10 seconds, stretch out both legs, one at a time, until your whole body is flat on the floor. Hold this long body stretch for a further 10 seconds. Sometimes I hold it for up to 3 minutes!

STEP FIVE ROUND-UP

So now you are eating properly and becoming more active. Stick with the things you have learnt in Steps One to Five until you are at a weight that's right for you. And if you remember to 'get moving' whenever you can as you shed your excess weight, you will soon become slim and fit.

Then move on to Step Six and find out how to consolidate everything you have learnt so that it will be easy for you to stay slim for life.

STEP SIX

Consolidate

From the moment you first picked up this book, you have been learning not just how to get slim, but how to *stay* slim for the rest of your life.

The ideas, thoughts, motivations and the insights and knowledge that this book has helped you to gain are those that will keep you on the right track in the years to come. And because you haven't been 'on a diet' as such, we have eliminated one of the greatest problems that most people meet when they do reach target weight at the end of a diet – how to get back to 'normal life' after being in 'dieting life'.

The way you have been eating to lose weight on the *Slim for Life* plan *is* normal eating. Once you are at the weight that feels right for you, you can simply carry on with your life, and your swops, and your new way of looking at things. There will be only one real change – *you can eat more.*

When you were losing weight, however slowly, you had to create a calorie deficit so that your body used its own fat stores for energy. Now that you no longer need a deficit, you will need enough food to maintain your new body weight, and this will inevitably mean eating more. So you just carry on eating in the pyramid fashion – or as near as you can get to it – but increasing the portion sizes.

Easy ways to weight maintenance

To give you an example of how simple the change is, many of you will have been eating, at least some of the time, around

25 triangles a day during your slimming campaign, using a pyramid-style diet like this:

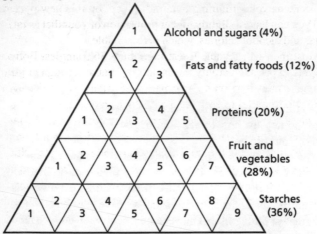

On your maintenance programme, you should be able to increase that to *at least* 36 triangles a day (remember, each triangle is worth 50 calories), which would look like this:

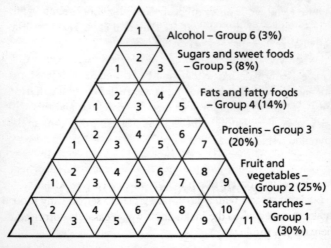

You can have 11 starch triangles a day; 9 fruit and vegetable; 7 protein; 5 fats; 3 sugars, and 1 alcohol. This balance is almost the same as your slimming pyramid, except on this new pyramid you can have a slightly higher proportion of your diet as fat, sugar and alcohol calories, which is reasonable.

Most men will be able to eat more than 36 triangles. Body weights, types and activity levels do vary, but as a rough guide I suggest men start on approximately 48 triangles, adding an extra two triangles to each level of the pyramid.

Unless you have been a long-term slimmer and chose to take the 'freestyle plan' on page 221 for more long-term flexibility, you will have been using the meal suggestions and recipes included in Step Four to form the basis of your slimming programme.

Now, to maintain your weight, you will want to add other foods and create your own menus. In order to help you do this, I have listed all the most popular food items with their triangle rating in the Food Charts starting on page 305. By using this list, you will find it easy to build your own pyramid-style diet, adding extra foods, creating your own recipes and using new foods as you wish.

The Food Charts group foods in exactly the same way as in the 36-triangle pyramid on the facing page so that you can easily see which 'tier' of the pyramid any particular food comes into and so tell how your day's pyramid is shaping up. You don't need to be precise – for instance, by always eating exactly 11 triangles of starchy foods a day. In fact, it would be very difficult to be absolutely precise. I'd like you to use the 36-triangle pyramid as nothing more than a guide. But as a matter of interest, it would be good now and then to have a day when you do check out more precisely what you're eating. To do this, draw up a blank 36-triangle pyramid and cross off each triangle when you have eaten food to that triangle value on each level.

I did this myself with a day's eating plan to see how my food intake matched up to the ideal, and I was pleasantly surprised. Here are my results:

A DAY'S MAINTENANCE EATING BASED ON THE PYRAMID 36-TRIANGLE SYSTEM

(△ = ¹/₂ triangle)

Day's low-fat spread for bread, scone, etc.: ▲ fats Group 4
Day's skimmed milk allowance for tea: ▲▲ protein Group 3

Breakfast

Average portion cereal: ▲▲ starches Group 1
1 large slice bread: ▲▲ starches Group 1
Pure fruit spread: △ fruit and vegetables Group 2
Skimmed milk extra to allowance: ▲ protein Group 3

Mid-morning snack

1 apple: ▲ fruit and vegetables Group 2

Lunch

Large portion home-made mixed vegetable and kidney bean soup: ▲▲▲▲ fruit and vegetables Group 2; ▲ fats Group 4
Large banana: ▲▲ fruit and vegetables Group 2

Teatime snack

1 wholemeal scone: ▲▲▲ starches Group 1; ▲ fats Group 4; ▲ sugars Group 5
1 glass orange juice: ▲ fruit and vegetables Group 2

Evening

Pasta, average serving: ▲▲▲▲▲▲ starches Group 1
Chicken and vegetable sauce: ▲▲ protein Group 3; ▲ fats Group 4; ▲ fruit and vegetables Group 2
Natural Greek yogurt: ▲▲ protein Group 3
Honey: △ sugars Group 5
Salad, large mixed: free + ▲ fruit and vegetables Group 2
1 glass wine: ▲▲ alcohol Group 6

When I totted up my triangles on the pyramid, it worked out very well – I had one triangle extra on both the starches and fruit and vegetables groups and, instead of using up all my sugars allowance, I had double alcohol allowance. Without carrying a notepad and calculator around with you most of the time you can't hope to eat a perfect pyramid every day. And, anyway, that is exactly the kind of obsessive behaviour you want to avoid. I've only shown you my day's eating plan to demonstrate that if you just 'think pyramid' then at least most of your mealtimes, you will be eating right and eating slim.

When you eat composite foods, especially ones you haven't cooked yourself, you may find it hard to know what you're eating, but you can take an educated guess. It may also help you to lump together Groups 4 and 5 and allow yourself up to 8 triangles a day of the sweet, fatty foods such as those listed on pages 314–17. Or, if you're fond of wine, like me, you could lump together the sugars Group 5 and the alcohol Group 6, allowing yourself up to 4 triangles a day for alcohol or sugars.

Remember, just keep 'thinking pyramid', cutting the fat and upping the carbohydrates, and even if you don't quite get there, you'll still be doing well. If you do this, it is almost impossible to eat too many calories and put on weight again.

PYRAMID MAGIC!

I'd like to give you one last example of what amazing things the pyramid idea can do for your waistline by demonstrating three different ways of serving up a 'beef and dessert' meal.

The first is an old-fashioned British-style roast lunch. The second is a 'halfway house' meal, based on a traditional British roast lunch but, by using all the 'swops' we learnt about in Steps Three and Four, we have cut the calories and fat drastically and are well on the way to giving the meal the pyramid feel. The third is a new-style pyramid meal, high on taste but even lower on fat and calories than meal two.

MEAL ONE:
OLD-FASHIONED-STYLE BRITISH LUNCH

Roast beef with vegetables

	Total calories	Fat calories	Grams of fat
110 g (4 oz) roast rib of beef (fat and lean)	383.0	285.0	31.7
2 chunks (150 g, 5½ oz) roast potatoes	235.0	65.0	7.2
Medium slice (50 g, 2 oz) Yorkshire pudding	105.0	45.0	5.0
Small portion (50 g, 2 oz) peas	27.0	3.1	0.35
Small portion (50 g, 2 oz) carrots	10.0	—	—
3 tablespoons pan gravy	45.0	36.0	4.0
2 teaspoons horseradish	10.0	2.0	0.2

Pudding

	Total calories	Fat calories	Grams of fat
Average slice (100 g, 3½ oz) apple pie	180.0	68.0	7.6
2 tablespoons double cream	135.0	130.0	14.5

Total weight of meal: 610 g

Total calories: 1,130

Total fat: 634 calories; 70.5 g; 6%

MEAL TWO: REDUCED-FAT-STYLE
BRITISH LUNCH

Roast beef with vegetables

	Total calories	Fat calories	Grams of fat
75 g (3 oz) lean cut roast beef (e.g., topside; no visible fat)	168.0	85.0	9.45
Medium (200 g, 7 oz) baked potato	170.0	2.0	0.2

Small slice (25 g, 1 oz)			
Yorkshire pudding	52.5	22.5	2.5
Medium portion (75 g, 3 oz) peas	31.0	2.7	0.3
Small portion (50 g, 2 oz) carrots	10.0	—	—
Small portion (50 g, 2 oz) broccoli	9.0	—	—
3–4 tablespoons gravy, fat-skimmed			
or from stock cube	10.0	trace	trace

Pudding

Average slice (150 g, 5¹/₂ oz)			
apple charlotte	203.0	40.5	4.5
2 tablespoons Greek yogurt	35.0	27.0	3.0

Total weight of meal: 700 g

Total calories: 688.5

Total fat: 179 calories; 20 g; 26%

MEAL THREE: NEW-STYLE PYRAMID MEAL

Chinese-style beef with rice

	Total calories	Fat calories	Grams of fat
60 g (2¹/₄ oz) lean-cut quick-fry			
beef, cut into strips	80.0	27.0	3.0
Spray of Fry Light cooking oil	18.0	18.0	2.0
25 g (1 oz) each green beans,			
broccoli, leek, carrot, courgette			
and mushrooms	38.0	trace	trace
2 teaspoons soya sauce	10.0	trace	trace
Knob ginger and sliced chilli	trace	trace	trace
Dash oyster sauce	8.0	trace	trace
25 ml (1 fl oz) beef stock			
from cube	10.0	trace	trace
70 g (2³/₄ oz) [dry weight]			
mixed long-grain and wild rice			
boiled with saffron	257.0	9.0	1.0

Dessert

	Total calories	Fat calories	Grams of fat
1 ripe fresh mango, sliced	110.0	—	—
1 tablespoon Greek yogurt	17.0	13.0	1.5

Total weight of meal: 615 g

Total calories: 550

Total fat: 67 calories; 7.5 g; 12%

As you can see, the total weight of the three meals is much the same, so you will have as much to eat on your plate whichever one you choose and not feel deprived or hungry. However, meal one is very high in calories and also has a very high fat content – 56 per cent – showing the wisdom of cutting down on the number of old-fashioned British-style meals. With meal two, just by making some simple 'swops', we have almost *halved* the calorie content and also *more than halved* the fat content! And, with meal three, by switching to the new pyramid-style meal, we have reduced both the calorie and fat content even further and still provided a tasty, appetising meal.

Easy, isn't it?! All you have to do for lifelong slimness, is to remember to make *swops* in what you eat, and build up a collection of new-style pyramid meals that you and your family will enjoy. International cuisine fits in perfectly with the pyramid philosophy – recipes from Mexico, India, China, Thailand, the Caribbean are all there just waiting for you to try. The choice is endless, so don't *ever* say keeping slim is boring.

Think pyramid most of the time and then you will be able to indulge in your own particular favourite treats when you want them, but the amazing thing is that the *longer* you eat pyramid-style, the *less* inclined you are to want the things that previously you found so alluring.

Feeling slim for life

So now you know what to eat and you know you can enjoy 'eating right' because you've proved it throughout your slimming campaign. But it is worth repeating a few of the most important things we learned in Step Three – the key pointers that will keep you eating and feeling like a slim person for always, because that is what you now are.

TIPS TO KEEP YOU SLIM FOR LIFE

- Remember, you are in control of what you put into your mouth – no-one else. It's your choice, but don't be obsessive or rigid in your control. Enjoy your food and feel relaxed about food. But never be afraid to say 'no' to the things you don't want.
- Don't feel guilty about enjoying hearty, tasty meals and don't feel guilty if occasionally you eat something that afterwards you wish you hadn't. Slim people eat all kinds of high- and low-calorie foods and stay slim because they take a 'swings and roundabouts' approach. You can do that too because you *are* a slim person.
- If you find difficulty in coping with certain areas of your eating habits, go back to Step Three and work through this or these areas again. There is no time limit on learning new ways to deal with your food intake.
- Remember, that you aren't perfect – no-one is.
- Be happy with sustainable goals. Don't try for too low a maintenance weight. Don't expect to look perfect – no-one does.
- Stay motivated and keep active.
- Listen to your body. It will let you know when you really are hungry.
- Eat slowly and enjoy your food.

- Remember, food isn't the most important thing in your life, even if it once was. Food is fuel to help you to a healthy body. You don't live to eat; you eat to live.

Write a list here of all the things that are important to you now:

....

....

....

....

....

STAY MOTIVATED

It is important to remind yourself now and then of all the ways your body, your mind and your life have improved since you began to lose weight. Go back now to Step One and read through all the motivators, even the ones that didn't apply to you at the time. Do you feel many of these benefits now? Which things can you work on to consolidate your success? What did you hope to achieve once you were slim? Isn't it time to start work on those ambitions now?

If everything is going on much as before, except that you feel slimmer and fitter and you like your body better – well, that's terrific too.

But in that case, can I offer you a motivator we didn't touch on in Step One, a motivator that will help everyone achieve long-term slimness. I would like you to get involved in a new campaign of mine – one that would ultimately result in me being rendered out of a job. I hope that, with your help, obesity in this country will eventually be wiped out, and that ill health through overweight and poor diet will be a thing of the past.

Sounds amazing? Well, maybe, but with your help, it could work. Turn to page 296 to see what you can do.

KEEP ACTIVE

People who keep themselves physically active find that they can eat plenty without putting on weight. If you combine a sensible pyramid-style of eating with a reasonable amount of activity, then you have the perfect way to control your weight for the rest of your life.

You can continue with the activity programme in Step Five, varying the amount you do from week to week according to what suits you.

To maintain fitness (as opposed to improving) most experts agree that two to three aerobic sessions and two strength/tone/flexibility sessions a week are all that's needed to keep you in shape.

But perhaps the single most important thing you can do to help maintain your new weight is to burn up extra calories each day by keeping as active as you can *outside* the confines of a formal exercise session. Your body needs to be used. Sitting around for most of the day and moving occasionally from bed to chair to car to desk to sofa to bed is not enough.

Give your body the attention it deserves throughout the day. All you need to do is to be aware of your body and to return a little to how your life might have been before TV, cars and labour-saving devices. Remember, every time you say 'yes' to a modern convenience that saves your body from moving or working, you're doing it a disfavour. Here are some ideas on getting more activity and movement into your everyday life:

- Think 'outdoors' as often as possible. Cycle or walk when you can (often it will be just as quick as waiting for a bus that never comes, or finding somewhere to park the car). Make the most of local facilities such as parks and nature trails.
- If you have a garden, spend more time in it. Gardening can be an absorbing and not too expensive hobby that anyone can enjoy.

- To give walking more of a purpose if you need one, consider walking a neighbour's dog or even a neighbour's baby.
- Don't just send your own children out to play – go with them and organise some active games like catch or rounders. Alternatively, take them swimming or roller-skating.
- Find out what clubs there are in your area that you could join. Your local council or library will have details.
- Try to increase the pace at which you do things, e.g., going up stairs, doing housework, carrying shopping, pushing a trolley, walking to work. Doing things faster means speeding up your metabolic rate and burning up more calories.
- Check your posture throughout the day. Whether you are standing or sitting, is your tummy pulled in, your bottom tucked in? Are your shoulders down and relaxed, rather than hunched?
- If you suffer from mid-afternoon sluggishness, don't fall asleep or eat a chocolate bar. If you feel drowsy or lack concentration during the day, a high-sugar, quickly absorbed snack will only end up making you feel worse. Instead, take a five-minute activity break: running up stairs or walking round the room or garden will put your body and brain back in good working order.
- Don't stay in bed longer than necessary to give you a refreshing sleep. Too much sleep can lower metabolism.
- Don't forget to breathe, preferably, good, fresh air. Like a fire, our bodies need oxygen to burn fuel (i.e. to convert food into energy and burn off calories). Whenever you get the chance, stand at an open window and breathe in deeply (not too deeply if you are unused to this as it will make you dizzy, but you'll soon improve). Always breathe calmly but deeply whatever you are doing.
- If you have long periods of standing or sitting, do some movements to get your circulation going again.

While sitting at desk or table: circle ankles; lift lower legs up and down and straighten legs out; flex heels to stretch calves; tighten and release thigh muscles; tighten and release buttock muscles; circle shoulders and gently turn head from left to right; gently pull head down to chest to release neck.

While standing in kitchen waiting for the kettle to boil: support yourself with one hand on work surface and do some leg sweeps (see page 262); stand with feet apart and knees bent and gently swing upper body down until fingers touch floor to release a tight back; clench buttock muscles; put one leg in front of the other and lift front heel off floor several times to exercise calf muscles.

By giving your body a series of mini workouts during the day you are doing a great deal to help keep it toned and supple, as well as burning off calories and preventing a build up of muscle tension.

Well, those are my ideas. I'm sure you can think of more. Write down here ten things you can do to build more activity into your life. Pick the ones that appeal to you from my list or choose your own.

....

....

....

....

....

....

....

....

....

....

Remember, if you want your body to be slim and to give you long-lasting, non-stop, uncomplaining service, treat it well, use it. You can't replace it!

Now see what you can change!

Over the last twenty years I have helped hundreds of thousands of people to lose weight through my books, magazine and newspaper columns. I hope that you are now one of them. But wouldn't it have been better if you hadn't had to slim because you hadn't put on the excess weight in the first place?

As we discussed in Step Two, there are many reasons why people put on too much weight. Most of those reasons can be summed up as 'outside influences' that made you eat too much of the wrong things and take too little exercise.

In order for you to lose weight I had to show you how to take control of your own body and cope with – or ignore – outside influences. Now that you are slim, you can go one better. Isn't it time to see what influence *you* can have on *others*? Not only on the people you know, but on the people and organisations who make the decisions that help keep us, as a nation, fat?

If we all campaigned determinedly enough, within a few generations we could have overweight, obesity, and the misery and ill health that they cause, licked for good.

ARE YOU A PARENT?

If you have children of your own, you should do everything you can to help them to a healthy lifestyle and way of eating. Even if they aren't overweight – as is the case with the majority of children – it is still important to get them into the habit of 'eating right'.

For most overweight people, it is the eating habits learned as children that are the root of their problems. And the reason why many children and teenagers who eat poor, high-fat, high-sugar, low-nutrient foods don't always have a weight problem is that they are at their most active during those years and are constantly growing. So they can support a very high-calorie intake without putting on weight. The small percentage who do get fat in childhood are probably very inactive and may have metabolic rates slower than average. Indeed, they may also eat more than average. But once children leave school, most of them tend to become much more inactive. Yet they carry on eating just as many of the high-fat, high-sugar foods as before, and gradually they put on weight.

In their twenties, many young adults will succumb to overweight as, like the majority of us, they give up almost all forms of exercise. It follows therefore that, rather than waiting until they are fat and then having to do something about it, the answer is to influence our children's diet and exercise habits right from the start.

There are very many things you can do to help if you are a parent, but first you need to know that growing children have one or two slightly different nutritional needs from their parents. Here are some general guidelines:

- Children under five years of age should never be given a very low-fat diet or too many fibre-rich foods. Children under two need whole milk to ensure adequate growth. Semi-skimmed milk can be gradually introduced from the age of two, provided the overall diet is adequate. From the age of five to eleven they can drink skimmed or semi-skimmed milk and eat more fibre.
- Growing children need plenty of protein and calcium in relation to their height, so the portions of lower-fat dairy products, lean meats and fish, poultry and pulses should certainly be as big as an adult woman's.
- Girls at puberty need plenty of iron (from lean red meat, leafy greens, dried fruits, sardines, whole grain cereals and wholemeal bread, for instance).

- Children who are slim and have voracious appetites should fill up on the healthy carbohydrates such as bread (not necessarily wholemeal), potatoes, pasta, rice and pulses, fresh and dried fruits.

If you want to ensure that your children grow up without the weight problems you have faced, here are the twelve best things you can do to influence that:

- Don't offer sweet treats as a reward for good behaviour or as consolation (for hurting themselves, being bored, etc.). Instead, offer fruit, or preferably, non-food rewards and palliatives. Don't give pre-school children sweets at all.
- Don't offer dessert to a child as a reward for eating up the main course. That gives them the idea that somehow the sweet course is worth more than the main course.
- Lead the way to healthier, slimmer eating by setting a good example. If children are brought up on a healthy diet based on the pyramid style of eating (but taking into account their specific nutritional needs), they will consider this the norm, and they will enjoy their food like any other child. Talk to your child about why it is important to give your body healthy fuel – they will understand and may be wiser than you give them credit for. They will also understand how the TV ads are influencing them.
- Make mealtimes as much fun and as relaxing as you can, with as much variety as you have time to offer. Remember, convenience foods don't have to be 'bad for you'. Pasta, baked beans, things on toast, and fruit-based desserts are all quick, easy and nutritious.
- Start feeding your children well as early on as possible. Eating tastes are simply habits built over a long period.
- Encourage your children to cook and take an interest in food. Don't let your children grow up thinking that a meal is just a ready-made dish you heat in a microwave. Help them to find interesting recipes in books and magazines

and encourage them to invent their own dishes based on their favourite foods. Have a weekly cook-in session instead of watching TV.

- Older children, who may resist change, can easily be given a slimmer, healthier diet by using all the 'swops' techniques you learnt in Steps Three and Four. Swop ordinary burgers for extra lean ones; crinkle chips for oven ones; butter for low-fat spread in sandwiches; mayonnaise or salad cream for reduced-calorie, low-fat dressings; and use lower-fat ice cream, cream and custard. Reduced-sugar items, like low-sugar baked beans and tomato ketchup and calorie-free squashes are useful too. But in the long term it is best to swop fizzy sugary drinks for more natural alternatives.

- Plan ahead to make sure older children who spend much time away from the house don't have to eat from takeaways or vending machines. Give them instant snacks to take with them, such as yogurt, fruit, fromage frais, dried fruit or packs of ready-shelled unsalted nuts (high in fat but a more nutritious alternative than many of the items they will find in a machine).

- Packed lunches may be preferable to giving children money to choose their own lunch (especially if their school doesn't have a good cafeteria). Nowadays, with insulated lunch boxes and wide-necked flasks, you can pack virtually anything, from soups in winter to yogurts in summer.

- If your children habitually leave food on their plates, get into the habit of giving them less, rather than making them eat up everything on their plate. So many overweight adults tell me that they were given over-large portions as children and made to eat everything up even when they were full. You can always give second helpings if children are still hungry, or fill them up with bread or fruit.

- Don't give sweet refined foods or commercial snacks if children are hungry between meals. Offer bread spread with Marmite or pure fruit spread; Crisprolls with vegetable pâté; yogurt; a banana; home-made popped corn; a home-made scone; some unsalted nuts, or sunflower seeds.

- When children are thirsty, offer them water or mineral water or, for a change, try fruit juice mixed with sparkling mineral water, or a milk shake made from semi-skimmed milk and a banana, whirred in a processor.

OUTSIDE INFLUENCES

In addition to the direct influence you can have over your children, there is plenty more you can do.

The latest research shows that children have up to 50 per cent influence on the foods parents put in their shopping trolley. And what the children want is usually directly related to what they have seen advertised on TV during children's television. These are the high added-value sugary, fatty, salty products like sugary breakfast cereals, sweets, crisp-type snacks and so on. Millions of pounds are spent each year advertising this kind of product to our children!

You can help to change this. Write to your MP and say you think food advertising during children's TV hours should be banned. Write to the advertising standards authority and tell them how you feel. Ask for their views. Write to the TV companies and tell them you will switch off if they don't modify their policy.

Write to the Department of Health and ask them what they are doing to improve the diet of our future generations. In fact they are addressing the problem with targets outlined in their recent White Paper, *The Health of the Nation* (1992), which aim to encourage manufacturers to produce foods containing less fat and sugar. However, if you write, it will help the Government to realise that if they want your vote they need to take action.

Your greatest influence is the fact that *you* are the person spending the money. Let your purse do the talking. The shops will soon stop stocking so many of the high-fat, high-sugar, high-calorie items if these don't move off the shelves. In turn, the manufacturers will quickly find healthier items to replace them with.

You can be heard, if your voice is strong enough. And if we *all* do it, our children won't be able to cry, 'Why can't I have that? Everyone else does ... '

Write to the food manufacturers and ask them what they are doing to reduce the fat and sugar content of their products (their addresses are often on the product packs or labels). If enough people do this, they will take notice.

Check out the standard of food in your child's school cafeteria (or at his future school). You are entitled to see a menu. If the standard of food doesn't look high, point this out to the head teacher. Get other parents interested and set up a meeting. Write direct to the caterers with your suggestions. Don't accept answers like, 'We just give the children what they want,' because what children want is appetising, filling food. They don't *want* highly refined, fatty, sugary foods – they simply eat these out of habit and often because there is no other choice. Don't just be negative though – always give your own suggestions as to how things could be improved.

Write to restaurant and takeaway chains – especially those designed to appeal to families and children – and ask for more thought to be given to producing lower-fat meals for children, and for less fatty, less sugary dessert alternatives. If you find places that *are* good, spread the word.

Write to the cookery editors of your favourite women's magazines and ask them to concentrate on providing more lower-fat, tasty recipes and always to provide an estimate of the fat and calorie content with each recipe. Ask them to ensure that not all their 'children's page' recipes are high fat, high sugar either.

Remember, you and your children are the consumers. You have the last word – if you will use it.

GET THEM MOVING, TOO!

All recent surveys conducted on the fitness and activity levels of our children and young adults show that they are nowhere near as active as they ought to be. Our children live in an age of TV and video games, of computers, and of diminishing emphasis placed on school sports and PE.

No wonder that research shows that by the time children are in their late teens, the majority are not even getting enough exercise to sustain moderate levels of fitness for their age.

Help your children to stay active throughout their life by helping them to good habits now. Here are some tips:

- When they are young, encourage them to play outside if you have a suitable area, rather than watching TV. Supervise them if necessary. If they don't have a safe place they can go to by themselves, you should take them out where they can be active. This depends largely on where you live and on your purse, but there is always something you can do if you are determined enough.

- Make full use of local council leisure facilities and find out what sports clubs there are in your area – your children will never know what they may be good at if they don't get the chance to try. Gymnastics, judo and orienteering clubs are all fun.

- Spend time watching your children when they are active, and talk to them to discover what they are naturally good at and what they like. Don't make children do sports they genuinely don't like. Not everyone will like or be good at everything, but there is always something they do like.

- Find out exactly what your children's school has to offer in the way of sports. If there doesn't seem enough emphasis on physical education, get together with other parents to discuss what can be done. If there is little out-of-hours sports activity, find out why. Perhaps with more volunteer help this could be changed.

- If there isn't much activity already organised in your area, why not start a club yourself? This can be as informal as you like – perhaps just a group of parents who have large gardens, each acting as host one session a week for simple games like rounders. Alternatively, you could hire a local hall or space for anything from tennis to five-a-side football. Or, if you have no space, you could form a rambling or cycling club.

- Encourage your older child to walk or cycle as a means of transport whenever feasible. Make sure your child is proficient at cycling by the age of ten and take him cycling whenever you can.

- If your child isn't very 'sporty' or doesn't enjoy competition, pick non-aggressive activities and avoid all talk of 'winning'. Help reticent children to be active. Again, walking and cycling are ideal, especially if you bring added interest to the activity, e.g., spotting wildlife or interesting buildings on a walk. Also try the activities that don't seem so much like 'formal exercise' or sport such as roller-skating, swimming or dancing.

- Talk to your children and make sure they understand why it is important to keep active.

WHAT ELSE CAN YOU DO?

If you don't have children of your own, perhaps you have children you know – younger brothers or sisters, nephews or nieces, grandchildren or neighbours' children. And you could offer to help in some of the above ways. Even if you don't know any children, you can still influence our future in a general manner by campaigning in some of the ways I've suggested in these pages. Perhaps you could offer to help all the hard-pressed parents and teachers who would do more if only they had the time. Volunteer to help out at after-school sports' sessions. If you have a talent, offer to teach. If you have transport, offer to take children to the pool or skating rink.

Everyone can do something to influence our future wellbeing. If we all help, we can look forward to the day when we don't spend most of our adult lives overweight and unfit.

Please write to me and tell me how you get on with our campaign. Tell me to whom you wrote, who you rang, who you saw, and what response you got. Tell me about setbacks and triumphs. And write and tell me if you have any *other* ideas and I'll do my best to publicise them.

And, of course, do write and tell me how you got on with your own *Slim for Life* programme. I'd really like to know what you thought of it.

Congratulations

Congratulations for getting this far! What we took together *was* six simple steps, but I didn't say they would be *easy*, did I?!

So give yourself a large pat on the back, and get on with your life – a life that will include good food and good exercise, but plenty more besides.

THE FOOD CHARTS

The charts will help you to follow a pyramid-style way of eating to maintain your new weight. The foods are grouped in the same way as in the 36-triangle pyramid that forms the 'blueprint' for your maintenance diet (see page 284).

They are:

Group 1: Starches group, including breads, crispbreads and bakery items; breakfast cereals; rice, grains and pasta; potatoes.
Aim for: approximately 11 triangles a day from this group.

Group 2: Fruit and vegetables group, including all fresh fruit; all fresh and frozen vegetables; fruit and vegetable juices; dried fruits and pulses.
Aim for: approximately 9 triangles a day from this group.

Group 3: Protein group, including low- to medium-fat cheeses; eggs; fish and seafood; low- to medium-fat meats; poultry; low- to medium-fat milk, yogurt and fromage frais products; vegetable proteins.
Aim for: approximately 7 triangles a day from this group.

Group 4: Fats group, including all fats and oils; oily dressings, nuts and snacks; all savoury high-fat and fried foods.
Aim for: 5 triangles a day from this group.

Group 5: Sugars and sweet items, including sweets and chocolate; cakes; biscuits and desserts.
Aim for: 3 triangles a day from this group.

Group 6: Alcohol.
Aim for: 1 triangle a day from this group, or amalgamate with the sugars Group 5, and aim for a total of 4 triangles a day for Groups 5 and 6.

Note: All triangle values are approximate, not exact – many values have been rounded up or down.

Group 1: Starches

BREADS, CRISPBREADS AND BAKERY ITEMS

All per 25 g (1 oz) unless otherwise stated.

No. of triangles

Bread

Brown, wheatgerm, white or wholemeal, per 40 g (1½ oz) slice from a large loaf, medium cut	2
French bread, brown or white	2
Petit pain, one whole	2
Pitta bread, white, one large	4
Pitta bread, wholemeal, one large	3
Pitta bread, one mini	2
Roll, one average	2½
Bap, one average	3

Crispbreads

Average rye crispbread, one	½
Crisproll, one	½

Bakery items

Crumpet, one	1½
Currant bun, one	3
English muffin, one	3
Malt loaf, 25 g (1 oz) slice	1½
Pancake, one average	2
Scone, one average	3
Teacake, one	3

BREAKFAST CEREALS

All per 25 g (1 oz) unless otherwise stated

All Bran	1½
Bran flakes or corn flakes	2
Fruit 'n' Fibre or muesli	2
Porridge oats, raw weight	2

No. of triangles

Porridge, made up with water, per 200 ml (7 fl oz) bowlful	2
Shredded Wheat, one	2
Weetabix, one	1½

RICE, GRAINS AND PASTA

Bulgar wheat or couscous, dry weight, per 25 g (1 oz)	2
Flour, white, wholemeal, soya or buckwheat, per 25 g (1 oz)	2
Pasta, all types, uncooked weight, per 25 g (1 oz)	2
Pasta, all types, boiled weight, per 100 g (3½ oz)	2
Pearl barley, dry weight, per 25 g (1 oz)	2
Rice, all types, dry weight, per 25 g (1 oz)	2
Rice, all types, boiled weight, per 100 g (3½ oz)	2
Semolina or polenta, dry weight, per 25 g (1 oz)	2

POTATOES

Baked, one average (225 g, 8 oz)	5
Boiled, per 100 g (4 oz)	1½
Mashed with 7 g (¼ oz) low-fat spread, per 100 g (3½ oz)	2½
Instant mashed, per 100 g (3½ oz)	2
Roast, 1 chunk (50 g, 2 oz)	2½
Sweet potato, baked or boiled, per 100 g (4 oz)	2
(for chips and crisps see Group 4)	

Group 2: Fruit and vegetables

DRIED FRUITS

All per 25 g (1 oz) unless otherwise stated

Apples, apricots, currants, figs, peaches, stoned prunes, raisins or sultanas	1
Stoned dates	1½

FRESH FRUIT

All per item unless otherwise stated	*No. of triangles*
Apple, dessert	1
Apple, cooking	1
Apricot, fresh, two	1
Banana, one small	1
Banana, one large	2
Blackberries, per 100 g (3½ oz)	1
Blackcurrants, per 100 g (3½ oz)	1
Cherries, per 100 g (3½ oz)	1
Damsons, per 100 g (3½ oz)	1
Dates, fresh, three	1
Fig, fresh	1
Gooseberries, dessert, per 100 g (3½ oz)	1
Gooseberries, cooking, per 100 g (3½ oz)	½
Grapefruit, one whole	1
Grapes, per 100 g (3½ oz)	1
Kiwifruit	1
Lemon, one whole	½
Lime, one whole	½
Mango	2
Melon, 200 g (7 oz) slice	1
Nectarine	1
Orange	1
Peach	1
Pear, one average	1
Pear, one large	1½
Pineapple, two slices	1
Plum, two dessert	1
Raspberries, per 100 g (3½ oz)	½
Rhubarb, per 100 g (3½ oz) [4 sticks]	½
Satsuma or tangerine	½
Strawberries, per 100 g (3½ oz)	½

FRUIT AND VEGETABLE JUICES

No. of triangles

All per 125 ml (4½ fl oz), average glass

Apple, grape, grapefruit, citrus, orange, pineapple or mixed	1
Mixed vegetable or tomato	½

NUTS

Chestnuts, shelled, per 25 g (1 oz)	1

(for all other nuts see Group 4)

PULSES

Baked beans in tomato sauce, canned, per 100 g (3½ oz)	1½
Butter beans, dry weight, per 25 g (1 oz)	1½
Butter beans, boiled or canned, per 100 g (3½ oz)	2
Chick peas, dry weight, per 25 g (1 oz)	2
Chick peas, boiled or canned, per 100 g (3½ oz)	3
Haricot beans, dry weight, per 25 g (1 oz)	1½
Kidney beans, dry weight, per 25 g (1 oz)	1½
Kidney beans, boiled or canned, per 100 g (3½ oz)	2
Lentils, brown or green, dry weight, per 25 g (1 oz)	1½
Lentils, brown or green, boiled, per 100 g (3½ oz)	2
Lentils, red, dry weight, per 25 g (1 oz)	2
Lentils, red, boiled, per 100 g (3 ½ oz)	2
Lentil soup, per 100 ml (3½ fl oz)	2
Split peas, dry weight, per 25 g (1 oz)	1½
Split peas, boiled, per 100 g (3½ oz)	2½

VEGETABLES

All per 100 g (3½ oz), raw or cooked without fat, unless otherwise stated

Artichoke, globe, one whole	1
Artichoke, Jerusalem	½

	No. of triangles
Asparagus, five spears	1/2
Aubergine	1/2
Avocado, half a medium	4
Beans, broad	1
Beans, French	1
Beans, runner	1/2
Beansprouts	1/2
Beetroot	1
Broccoli	1/2
Brussels sprouts	1/2
Cabbage, all types	1/2
Carrots	1/2
Cauliflower	1/2
Celeriac	1/2
Celery	1/2
Chicory	1/2
Chinese leaves and Pak Choi	1/2
Corn on the cob, one medium	2
Courgettes	1/2
Cucumber	1/2
Leeks	1/2
Lettuce, all types	1/2
Marrow	1/2
Mushrooms	1/2
Mustard and cress	1/2
Onion, one large	1
Onion, one small	1/2
Onion, spring, one bunch	1/2
Parsnip	1
Peas	1
Pepper, green	1/2
Pepper, red or yellow	1
Radish	1/2
Spinach	1/2

	No. of triangles
Swede	1/2
Sweetcorn kernels	2
Tomato, one large	1/2
Turnip	1/2
Watercress	1/2

Group 3: Proteins

CHEESES

Brie, per 25 g (1 oz)	1½
Camembert, per 25 g (1 oz)	1½
Cheddar-style, half-fat, per 25 g (1 oz)	1½
Cottage, per 100 g (3½ oz)	2
Cottage, diet, per 100 g (3½ oz)	1½
Edam, half-fat type, per 25 g (1 oz)	1½
Low-fat soft cheese, e.g., Shape, per 40 g (1½ oz)	1
Mozzarella, per 25 g (1 oz)	1½
Quark low-fat, per 100 g (3½ oz)	2½
Reduced-fat cheese spread, per 25 g (1 oz)	1

EGGS

Size 1 or 2, each	2
Size 3 or 4, each	1½
Size 3 egg, one, dry-fried	2
Size 3 egg, two, scrambled with 7 g (¼ oz) low-fat spread and dash skimmed milk	4

FISH AND SEAFOOD

Fish

Cod or coley or haddock fillet, per 100 g (3½ oz)	1½
Halibut steak or plaice fillet, per 100 g (3½ oz)	2

	No. of triangles
Haddock, smoked fillet, per 100 g (3½ oz)	2
Herring, grilled, per 100 g (3½ oz)	4
Kipper, grilled, per 100 g (3½ oz)	4
Monkfish, per 100 g (3½ oz)	1½
Pilchards in tomato sauce, per 100 g (3½ oz)	3
Salmon, fresh fillet, per 100 g (3½ oz)	4
Salmon, canned, drained, per 100 g (3½ oz)	3
Salmon, smoked, per 50 g (2 oz)	1½
Trout, rainbow fillet, per 100 g (3½ oz)	3
Tuna steak, fresh, per 100 g (3½ oz)	3
Tuna canned in brine, drained, per 100 g (3½ oz)	2
Tuna canned in oil, drained, per 100 g (3½ oz)	2½
Fishcake, one, grilled	2
Fish fingers, one, grilled	1
Fish, frozen crumbed portion, baked or grilled, one	4

Seafood
All per 100 g (3½ oz), shelled or dressed weight

Crab	2½
Prawns	2
Mussels	2
Scallops	2
Squid	1½

MEAT AND POULTRY

All per 100 g (3½ oz) unless otherwise stated

Meat

Beef, extra-lean, minced	4
Beef, steak, no visible fat	4
Beef, topside, roast	3
Beef, roast rib, including fat	5
Beef, roast rib, fat removed	4
Beefburger, lean, grilled, 1 × 50 g (2 oz)	2

	No. of triangles
Corned beef	4
Ham, extra-lean	2½
Kidneys, lamb's, each	1
Lamb, leg, roast, lean only	4
Lamb chop, extra-lean, trimmed, grilled, one	3
Liver, grilled	3½
Pork, roast, lean only	3½
Pork fillet, raw	3½
Rabbit, flesh only	3
Sausages, low-fat, grilled, per chipolata	1
Veal	2

Poultry and game

Chicken, meat only (no skin)	3
Chicken, roast, meat and skin	4
Duck, roast, lean only	4
Turkey, roast or fillet	2
Venison	4

MILK, YOGURT AND FROMAGE FRAIS

Milk, semi-skimmed, per 100 ml (3½ fl oz)	1
Milk, skimmed, per 150 ml (5½ fl oz)	1
Milk, soya, per 150 ml (5½ fl oz)	1
Yogurt, diet fruit, per tub	1
Yogurt, fruit, low-fat, per 100 ml (3½ fl oz)	2
Yogurt, Greek cow's, strained, per 100 ml (3½ fl oz)	3
Yogurt, Greek ewe's, per 100 ml (3½ fl oz)	2
Yogurt, natural low-fat, per 100 ml (3½ fl oz)	1
Yogurt, whole milk, per 100 ml (3½ fl oz)	3
Fromage frais, diet fruit, per tub	1
Fromage frais, natural, 0% fat, per 100 ml (3 ½ fl oz)	1
Fromage frais, natural, 8% fat, per 100 ml (3½ fl oz)	2½

VEGETABLE PROTEINS

	No. of triangles
Quorn, per 100 g (3½ oz)	1½
Tofu, per 100 g (3½ oz)	1½
TVP (soya mince), per 100 g (3½ oz), reconstituted weight	1½

Group 4: Fats

FATS AND OILS

All per 25 g (1 oz) unless otherwise stated

Butter	4
Margarine	4
Polyunsaturated margarine	4
Low-fat spread	2
Very low-fat spread	1½
Oil, all types	5
Oil, 1 tablespoon	2½

DRESSINGS

All per tablespoon (15 ml, ½ fl oz)

French dressing	2
Mayonnaise	2
Mayonnaise, reduced-calorie	1
Salad cream	1

CHEESES

All per 25 g (1 oz)

Mature Cheddar	2
Cream cheese, full-fat	2½
Stilton	2½
Blue Brie	2½

CREAM AND MILK

	No. of triangles
Single, per 25 ml (1 fl oz)	1
Double, per 25 ml (1 fl oz)	2
Double, half-fat, per 25 ml (1 fl oz)	1
Whipped, per tablespoon	1
Milk, whole, per 75 ml (3 fl oz)	1
Milk, whole, per average glass	3½

FRIED FOODS

Egg size 3, fried, one,	3
Fish, deep-fried in batter, one average portion	6–8
Chips, per 100 g (3½ oz)	5
Oven chips, per 100 g (3½ oz)	3½

MEAT

Bacon, back, average grilled, one slice	3
Bacon, back, trimmed, grilled, one slice	2
Bacon, streaky, grilled, one slice	3
Beef, average minced, per 100 g (3½ oz)	5
Duck, roast, including skin, per 100 g (3½ oz)	7
Lamb shoulder, roast, per 100 g (3½ oz)	6
Lamb chop, including fat, one average	7
Liver sausage, per 50 g (2 oz)	3
Luncheon meat, per 50 g (2 oz)	3
Salami, per 50 g (2 oz)	5
Sausages, beef or pork, grilled, one large	2½
Frankfurter, one	1
Tongue, per 50 g (2 oz)	2

NUTS AND SNACKS

	No. of triangles
All per 25 g (1 oz) shelled weight	
Almonds or brazils	3
Hazelnuts	2
Peanuts or peanut butter	3
Walnuts	2½
Crisps, standard	2½
Crisps, lower fat	2

PASTRY ITEMS

Filo pastry, per 25 g (1 oz)	1½
Flaky pastry, per 25 g (1 oz)	3
Shortcrust pastry, per 25 g (1 oz)	2½
Meat pie, one individual	10
Pasty, Cornish, one	9
Pork pie, one individual, 140 g (5 oz)	11

Group 5: Sugars and sweet items

BISCUITS, CONFECTIONERY AND SOFT DRINKS

Biscuits, digestive, each	1½
Biscuits, chocolate, each	2
Cake, fruit, 50 g (2 oz) slice	3
Cake, sponge, 50 g (2 oz) slice	3
Cheesecake, 75 g (3 oz) slice	6
Chocolate, milk or plain, per 25 g (1 oz)	3
Cola, one can	2½
Croissant, one small	3
Doughnut, jam, one	4½

	No. of triangles
Eclair, chocolate, one	3
Fruit pie, 125 g (4¹/₂ oz) portion	7
Ice cream, 50 g (2 oz) portion	2
Jam or honey, two teaspoons	1
Lemonade, one can	2
Pastry, Danish, one	7
Sugar, any kind, one teaspoon	¹/₂
Sweets, boiled, per 25 g (1 oz)	2
Toffees, per 25 g (1 oz)	2

Group 6: Alcohol

Beer, per 275 ml (¹/₂ pint)	2
Lager, per 275 ml (¹/₂ pint)	2
Extra-strong lager, per 275 ml (¹/₂ pint)	3
Spirits, all, one measure	1
Stout, per 275 ml (¹/₂ pint)	2
Wine, medium or dry, 140 ml (5 fl oz) glass	2
Wine, sweet, 140 ml (5 fl oz) glass	3
Champagne, 140 ml (5 fl oz) glass	3